# A HAPPIER HOUR

# A HAPPIER HOUR

## Rebecca Weller

Mod By Dom ~ Australia

A HAPPIER HOUR

Cover and Interior Design by Dominic Garczynski
Cover Photography by Royden Monteiro

ISBN: 9780994602381
Digital ISBN: 9780994602312
Paperback ISBN: 9780994602305
Audiobook ISBN: 9780994602343

For anyone struggling with similar challenges.
You are loved, and you are not alone.

And for Dom, who never let me forget it.

# ONE

A blaze of sunlight snuck its way through a gap in the blinds, drilling directly into my eyelids, punishing me. Desperately, I held them closed. The pain arrived a split-second later; loud and brimming with intent, like a diva making her dramatic entrance. My skull felt like it was cracking from the inside, and every breath caused my body to tremble and ache. Even my hair hurt. Every strand of it throbbed in agony, sending a thumping SOS to my brain.

Slowly, carefully, I opened one eye. The pain intensified. I was still in last night's outfit, and judging by the way my eyelashes were stuck together, last night's makeup as well. *What the hell.*

I was so thirsty, I felt like I could drink all the water in all the oceans of the world. Thankfully, Dominic had placed a glass of water on my bedside table, although I knew I didn't deserve it. I gulped it greedily and was immediately hit with a wave of nausea.

I fell out of bed and scrambled through my handbag, as I'd done a thousand times before, desperately hoping I hadn't lost anything. In the pale morning light, I found my keys, my purse, my... *Oh God.* My phone was missing. I tried to piece together the night before. Did Dom simply put it somewhere for safekeeping? I scoured the apartment with bleary eyes. No such luck.

Taking a deep, shaky breath, I tip-toed back to our bedroom. I really didn't want to wake him, especially not with this news. A conversation we'd had a few weeks earlier played in my head, taunting me. "You need to put a security code on your phone," he lectured, "so that it's locked, if you ever lose it." Only, I hadn't quite gotten around to it yet.

I carefully climbed back into bed and tapped his shoulder.

"Call your parents," he sighed, after I told him the situation. "See if it's at the hotel."

I left him in bed, hoping he wasn't too mad. In the kitchen, I grabbed his phone and switched it on. My family were scheduled on an early morning flight to Bali, and I felt increasingly stressed out, hoping I wouldn't miss them before they left their hotel.

His phone flashed to life with a loud beep, signalling one voicemail message. I held my breath as it connected. A few seconds later, I heard my Step-Dad's voice, "Hey Bec, we found your phone. We'll leave it with reception when we check out, okay. We'll see you in a couple of weeks. Love you."

I let out a huge sigh of relief, causing my body to shudder again. I poured myself another glass of water and attempted to drink the whole thing. My body accepted three-quarters of it before calling a strike.

I crept back into the bedroom. Maybe if Dom had gone back to sleep, he'd forget all about this.

"Well?" he asked.

"Yep, they found it," I whispered, crawling back into bed. "So I guess I'll drive out there later today."

He sighed again and climbed out of bed. I waited for him to say something, but he didn't. Instead, he headed for the shower, leaving me alone with my thoughts. The place I was most afraid to be.

I frantically tried to remember the events of the night before. My parents, sister, and her family, had managed to arrange an early check-in at a hotel near the airport. We'd originally planned to meet them there for dinner and drinks, but impatient to join the festivities, I asked my boss if I could leave at lunchtime, and scooted out the door. I sent Dom a text message, letting him know I was heading over earlier than planned, and he agreed to meet us there later. As always, my family popped the champagne the second I arrived.

And that's where my memory gets hazy. I vaguely remember Dom sending a text message to let me know he was still stuck at work, and "please don't drink too much."

A blur of time passing. Two more bottles? Maybe three? Then Dom arriving and encouraging us to order dinner, urging me to "please eat something." But no doubt the damage was already done.

It was only now, in the cold light of morning, that I realised how ridiculous the whole scene must have looked. Dom and I had been living together for six months, and in love for a year. By all accounts, we were still in the honeymoon phase. Only, his patience with my drinking antics was wearing dangerously thin, and I knew it.

He returned from the shower and dressed in silence. He obviously wasn't ready to talk to me, so I figured it best to wait a while. Probably best to wash off the smell of alcohol first.

In the shower, I was still trembling. What kind of woman can't remember how she got home, and loses her phone, past the age of twenty-five? *A big, old lush, that's who.* Under the steaming hot water, I closed my eyes and held my breath, attempting to wash the hateful thoughts from my mind. It was no use. I wanted to collapse onto the shower floor and sob, but my body ached too much. *Why the hell did I keep doing this to myself?*

When I finally got out of the shower, Dom was gone.

~

An 8am meeting meant I had to be at work before I could even contemplate retrieving my phone.

As I drove into the carpark closest to my office, I prayed

I'd make it through the meeting without throwing up or passing out.

I managed. *Just.*

The second the meeting was over, I vanished; stealthily making my way along the outer hallways, back to the privacy of my car. My hands were still trembling as I turned the key in the ignition. As I drove, I cranked the radio up and tried not to think about anything besides getting there in one piece.

Twenty minutes later, I pulled into the hotel carpark, happy to discover that my car was amongst only half a dozen or so. I prayed that the hotel wouldn't be busy. I couldn't handle more eyes on me right now.

I held my throbbing head as high as I could manage. Taking a deep breath, I walked into the lobby. To my utter relief, it was deserted. Just one man stood behind the reception desk.

"Hi. Um. My family found my phone last night and left it here for me to pick up?" I said, trying to breathe as little as possible so he wouldn't smell my hangover. Was he on duty last night? Did he see me leave in my drunken state? '*That boozy woman came in to get her phone,*' he'd tell the rest of the staff later, '*and did she ever stink!*' And they'd all fall about laughing. Probably.

The huge clock on the wall slowed down, the loud tick of each passing second drilling itself into my psyche. Finally, after an eternity, he returned and handed it over, putting me out of my misery. As I turned to make a hasty exit, a loud crack of thunder shook the building. A second later, the skies opened and rain bucketed down, mirroring my mood. *Great.* Phone in hand, I ran back to the car as fast as my fragile state would allow, jumped in, and checked my text messages.

There was just one. Received from Dom at 9:49am, "How about I just hand in my resignation tomorrow?"

I smiled, grateful that his mind had moved on to things other than how disappointed he was in me. Over the past few months, we'd been talking about wanting to resign from our corporate careers. Neither of us were flourishing in our current roles, and our imaginations had been captured by tales of people launching themselves into entrepreneurship and supporting themselves with their skills and talents.

I'd mentioned the whole crazy idea to my family the night before, after Dom had sent me a half-joking text: "How about this time next month we hand in our resignations? I'm drowning in this role, and Jack wants to quit this week! I've got some savings that can cover rent for a few months."

Champagne in hand, I'd texted him back: "haha, definitely an option! I have some savings too. Let's talk strategy!"

While my sister thought I was just being drunk and ridiculous, my parents seemed surprisingly supportive. Then again, perhaps they were just humouring me.

I stared out the windscreen at the passing traffic. I noticed the damp, musty smell that older cars get when it rains, and I couldn't will myself to move. How had I gotten to the point of just disappearing from work? Not only was I thirty-eight years old and hungover as hell, now I was unreliable to boot. I checked the time on the dashboard. 11:13am. I typed a new message to Dom: "I'm sitting in the hotel carpark. I left the office an hour ago and didn't tell anyone I was leaving. I don't want to go back!"

Two seconds later, my phone buzzed with his reply. "Come meet me for lunch."

In a daze, I started the car and headed to the café nearest his office.

I arrived to find it busier than I'd hoped, but I manoeuvred my way through the lunchtime crowd to find a cosy table near the back. From my vantage point, I could see into the kitchen. The sight and smell of sizzling food reminded me just how hungry I was.

I texted Dom, and he arrived in a heartbeat. I watched as he strode through the café. *God, he was sexy.* He was a man on a mission; his height only adding to the effect. It was intoxicating.

"So," he said, smiling and hanging his coat on the back of his chair. "I was serious about my text. Let's do it. Tomorrow."

A current of emotions ran through me, providing a welcome reprieve from my hangover. My head spun with a thousand conflicting thoughts. "Seriously?" I said. "Are we really doing this?"

Dom searched my face, reading my expression. He smiled, taking my hands in his. "Yes."

~

Over breakfast the next morning, I double-checked with Dom. "So we're really doing this?" My work day started an hour earlier than his, so I wanted to be sure—really sure— he wasn't just teasing me, before I did something I'd regret.

"We're really doing it!" he beamed, crunching on a piece of toast.

"Okay!" I yelped, grabbing my bag and closing the front door behind me.

My office was only a fifteen-minute walk away. As I ambled along the tree lined streets, I thought about how fabulously spontaneous this whole plan was.

The minute I got to my desk, I texted Dom, "Okay, this is it! I'm doing it. You better do it too!"

I switched on my computer while I waited for final confirmation. Two minutes later, my phone buzzed with his reply, "I'm doing it!"

We'd printed our letters of resignation the night before, and my hand shook as I carried it across the office to see my boss. I always hated this part.

"Hi Sean. Do you have a moment?" I said, tapping on his open office door.

"Sure," he replied, looking up from his computer. "What's up?"

As he watched me close the door behind me, his smile faded. "Oh, no. What's happened?" he asked.

We were working on a multi-billion dollar project, and the work was becoming increasingly chaotic as the company restructured itself. As the manager of our rapidly dwindling Project Controls team, Sean was no stranger to office drama.

I sat down, took a deep breath, and launched in. "I want to start by saying you are a wonderful boss and I've loved working for you..." I paused for a second. It had all tumbled out of me so quickly, I wondered if he'd understood any of it.

"Oh, no," he groaned, pulling a *here-we-go* face.

"Afraid so," I said, handing him the letter, my heartbeat pounding in my ears.

He sighed loudly. "Where are you going?" The city was alive with projects and positions, and it was only natural he'd want to know.

"I'm going to work for myself!" I said out loud for the very first time, and giggled. The concept still seemed so foreign and surreal.

"Hey... What?" His pained expression was replaced with curiosity.

"I'm going to be a health coach," I explained. "See, a couple of years ago, I started this little hobby food blog..."

"Show me!" he demanded, grinning and pointing towards his computer.

And I thought, *this is why everyone loves him.*

~

Leaving Sean reeling in his office, I floated back to my desk and looked around at my team mates, all hard at work in their cubicles. I wondered whether I should break the news to them, or tell my girlfriends first. It was so quiet in the office that morning. Soft key strokes and the occasional cough reverberated around the stillness. Even if I whispered the news, everyone on our floor would be sure to hear.

Embarrassed to make a fuss, I decided to tell to my girlfriends first. I'd been with the company for eight years and had made a great circle of friends in other departments. I poked a key, waking my computer. Still nervous with excitement, I fired off a quick email telling them about not only my resignation, but Dom's too.

A heartbeat later, my phone rang. "But how will you *live?!*" Chloé almost shouted down the line, and I stifled a giggle. I loved dramatic friends.

"I've got some savings, honey, and Dom does too. If we're frugal, we might have enough to cover our living expenses for six months. We're just going to give it a go, and see what happens. It's an *experiment*," I told her.

"But… Can't *one* of you stay employed?" she wailed.

"We thought about it, we really did," I nodded and smiled, even though she couldn't see me. "But we want to do this together."

Secretly, I hoped that by starting our own business, I'd naturally—*magically*—drink less. Dom was a good influence, and I'd convinced myself that my drinking was only escalating along with the stress in my current role. I tried not to think about how much I drank when I was in a different department, or during my roles in Sydney, or London. Because if I was honest, my drinking style now wasn't remarkably different to my drinking style when I was a teenager. Fast, copious, and relentless.

Only now, I prayed I'd have a reason to stop.

# TWO

When I discovered, at age sixteen, that alcohol could magically transform me into the confident and outgoing girl I longed to be, I fell in love with it. Never mind that it regularly kicked my ass, made me do and say stupid things, and stole my self-worth. Most of the time (okay, at least half of the time), it made me feel glamorous, fun, and hilarious. Before I'd even turned eighteen, I couldn't imagine a social life without it.

It was just sips at first. Cider, summer wine, and alcopops at weekend parties. Midori and lemonade if we managed to sneak into a bar. A girl drinking girly drinks, playing at being a grown-up.

Like a holiday romance, it escalated quickly. Sips became gulps. Gulps became cans and bottles skulled in corners and behind doors. Dutch Courage became recklessness. Wild abandon grew into annihilation.

Other girls seemed to have an 'off' switch that wasn't installed in me. They'd feel sick, or throw up, and take that as a sign that they should stop. Not me. While I was drinking, I always felt like I was having the time of my life, so I did what any party girl would do; I kept going. I loved the feeling of the room spinning. Like I was on a magical merry-go-round; fairy lights whirling around me, far away from the relentless thoughts and anxiety in my head.

Overdrinking relieved my overthinking, and God help the poor soul who tried to pry the bottle from my vice-like grip.

High School parties were a mess for me. Boys, blackouts, and embarrassment.

Technical college gave me a clean slate. A fresh start.

It was there, in one of my classes, that I met my first love. Five years later, we were engaged and living in a house we'd built in the suburbs. But I wasn't happy, and my drinking had only intensified. So I did the only thing I could think of. I broke up with him, amidst a flood of tears and a hangover, on New Years Day, 1999.

"You won't find what you're looking for," he told me, as he watched me pack. Which might have worried me, if I'd even had a single clue what I was looking for.

Aged twenty-three, I boarded a plane to London with no return ticket.

~

In London, I felt liberated. Free to start again with a clean slate.

My school friend Kate picked me up from Heathrow Airport. Exhausted from the long-haul flight, it was so good to see a familiar face. We squealed as we hugged hello, and she helped me carry one of my heavy suitcases to the tube station.

Kate had been living in London for a year or so, and she'd arranged a place for me in her large share house in Finsbury Park. The house was run by an older Australian couple, and consisted of ten bedrooms spread over three floors. The lower floor, partially sunken into the ground, contained the kitchen and a large living room, and each floor held a small bathroom.

"Make sure you get up early if you want a shower in the morning," Kate advised me, as we lugged my suitcases past the first bathroom door. "With twenty-four housemates, it can be a bit of a wait."

As we walked along the narrow corridor, I peeked past bedroom doors that had been left open. Most rooms held a single set of bunkbeds or a double bed. The rooms were tiny, but seemed comfortable enough.

"You're in bedroom ten," Kate told me, as we struggled our way up the creaky stairs. "Right up the top." Before I'd arrived, she'd warned me that the bedroom I was assigned to held four beds.

"Okay," I giggled, following her lead.

After living in my own house for such a long time, I was nervous about meeting my three roommates. Four strangers, sharing a bedroom. What if they snored? What if *I* did? I reassured myself that it was, at worst, a temporary arrangement. I'd submitted a request to be transferred to a smaller bedroom as soon as one became available.

*Plus,* I reasoned, *I can always move to another apartment or something, if I don't like it.*

That night, I met my three roommates. Kate had already gone back to her bedroom when they suggested we crack open a bottle of vodka to celebrate our new living arrangements.

My first night, and they were already suggesting drinks. *Oh, I had a feeling I was going to like it here.*

And drink we did. Excited about this fresh start and buoyed by our intoxicated intimacy, I blurted out private details that I'd regret the following day. Then I promptly fell off my top bunk bed, head-first into the floor. While my roommates rushed downstairs to find frozen peas, I laughed and blamed it on the jet lag. Jet lag with vodka chaser.

~

I found contract work easily, despite the 'Aussie accent' I didn't realise I had. My time working for a recruitment agency in Perth meant the London agencies trusted me and quickly sent me for assignments all over the city. I was placed in the investment banking industry, which suited me just fine. They had huge entertainment budgets, which meant more opportunities for drinking.

"You Aussie girls are so brash," one of my colleagues told me one day.

"Brash?" I asked, pulling a face like a puppy when you hide its tennis ball.

"Reckless," he elaborated.

I certainly didn't feel reckless normally, but I loved that alcohol made me feel that way. Wild, dangerous and exciting. It seemed so much more appealing than my sober mode of operation; timid, anxious and unsure of myself.

The whole travelling lifestyle suited me as well. No long-term responsibilities, no demands to get serious about myself or my future. Between having twenty-three housemates, and an office full of colleagues who were always up for a pint and a laugh, I found myself drinking more than ever.

London was wild. It was a different culture here. Spending lunch breaks in the pub was actively encouraged. At night, the pubs closed at 11pm, so there was always the feeling that you had to rush. *Get one more round in, quick, before the final bell.* Thursdays nights were favoured in particular. As my colleagues often joked, "So we can nurse our hangovers on company time."

I put on a lot of weight that year, although I was too drunk to notice until one fine morning when I was getting ready for work and split my skirt straight up the back hem. It was then that I realised I'd been wearing the same skirt for weeks, as it was the only one that still fit my growing frame. Evidently I was hoping that if I ignored the issue, I'd somehow—magically—fit back into the rest of my wardrobe. In desperation, I woke my room mate to ask if I could borrow something of hers, and vowed to cut back on the muffins and cheesy sandwiches. Not the alcohol, of course. Never the drink.

The work assignments were fairly easy, and on my weeks off, I headed abroad to see places I'd only ever dreamt about. I travelled with new friends to France, Spain, Scotland, Ireland, Switzerland, Belgium, New York, South Africa, and the Greek Islands. Every new place was a chance to see how the locals partied.

For the most part, living in London was a great adventure; deliciously liberating after being mortgage-ridden in a too-serious, too-young, relationship. But every once in a while, I experienced a homesickness that almost drowned me in grief. It would sneak up on me, tapping me on the shoulder when I was at my most vulnerable, usually while I was nursing a hideous hangover. I'd been living in London for almost three years, and although it had started out exciting, as time went on, I found myself drinking more and growing increasingly unhappy.

~

My friend Heather and I were on a flight back to London from Athens when the planes hit the Twin Towers in New York on September 11th, 2001. Nobody said a word about it to us as we disembarked our plane, or as we waited by the baggage carousel, or as we cleared customs. When we descended into the underground tube station at Heathrow and headed for home, we noticed that it was eerily empty. The heaving mass of people usually jammed into the carriages on a Tuesday night was strangely missing. Still, we had no clue.

It was only when we walked into our living room that we suspected something was up. Six of our housemates were glued to the television screen in silence; an incredibly rare phenomenon. I looked at Heather. She shrugged. *It must be one heck of a movie.*

"What are you watching?" I asked.

Six pairs of eyes slowly turned to look at me.

"What are we watching? Where the fuck have you two been!" our housemate Aaron boomed, flinging a newspaper towards us.

"Greece," I mumbled, as I picked up the newspaper and stared at the front page. "What the...?" I looked back at him, demanding an explanation. Everyone else remained silent.

"Here, watch this," he finally sighed, clicking the remote control to switch to a 24-hour news channel. We watched wide-eyed as the whole horrific scene was replayed in bold technicolour.

"Oh my God," I whispered.

"Yep," nodded Aaron. "They've grounded all planes, everywhere. We were sent home early from work. People are *freaking the fuck out.*"

"So... We... What? Do we go to work tomorrow?" I

asked in bewilderment.

"Fuck knows!" he said, standing to leave the room. "Call your boss."

Instead, I called my family to let them know I was safely back in London. Although, to be honest, since I worked in the central financial district, I wasn't sure exactly how safe that was.

I didn't have my boss's number, so the next morning I headed to work, and breathed a huge sigh of relief to see other people at Liverpool Street station. Less people than usual, but people, nonetheless.

The next few weeks were a mess of anthrax scares, evacuations, and desperately trying to find out if all members of our Manhattan office were safe and accounted for. Several times as I walked to work, I burst into tears, frightened for the state of the world.

Our team still went for drinks, but there was a surreal and sombre quality to those nights, as though we knew we were all standing on quicksand. I began buying an extra bottle of wine on my way home each night, determined to drink myself into a cosy state of numbness that remained just out of reach.

I wanted to go home.

On a still and frosty day in December 2001, aged twenty-six, I boarded a plane back to Australia.

~

Suspecting that Perth would feel too quiet for me after

London life, I convinced my friend Jess to move to Sydney with me. Jess was originally from New Zealand and we'd worked together in London. Neither of us had visited Sydney for any extended period of time, but we were young and free, and it seemed like an exciting place to start a new adventure.

I quickly landed a role in the head office of one of Australia's largest banks, right in the heart of the city. Jess and I found ourselves a small apartment in North Bondi, and I was excited about the prospect of working and partying in the city all week, then relaxing on the beach all weekend. *Talk about living the Sydney lifestyle!*

I was excited to find that the culture in the Australian investment banking industry was much the same as it had been in London. Our department had a huge budget for entertaining, and every other week we were treated to champagne and cocktail celebrations in some of the city's most extravagant bars. Friday lunchtime drinks were the norm, as were spontaneous mid-week drinking sessions.

In spite of all the free bar tabs and functions, I still managed to spend a huge portion of my wages on drinking. Late-night rounds, lunch sessions, taxi fares. Not to mention, replacing lost purses, earrings, phones and jackets.

Jess found a position in a nearby investment bank and we often met up after work. She'd come out with my colleagues, or I'd go out with hers. We were young, single, and always up for a great night out. Sometimes we met cute guys and stayed out even later than usual.

"I've been counting. How many of those things do you think you've had tonight?" asked one such guy, gesturing towards our drinks, on a particularly late night in a city bar.

We glanced down at the cider bottles in our hands, and then at each other. "Um… nine?" Jess offered.

"Nope," he said, pausing for effect. "Fourteen!" he finally yelled, roaring with laughter. "You chicks sure can drink!"

"No! Not fourteen!" I protested, shaking my head. Determined to prove he was exaggerating, Jess and I began counting, retracing our steps throughout the night. Six, eight, ten, twelve… *Damn*, he was right.

Horrified, Jess and I promptly exited the bar, leaving him and his friend behind. We walked to a late-night junk food place down the road and promised each other we'd slow down on the drinking. *London must have increased our tolerance*, we reasoned. It was time to cut back to more ladylike levels.

My steely determination lasted exactly seven days. The following Friday night, I drank so much that I spent the entire next day throwing up. I'd spent entire days hungover and vomiting before, but this was a new level of pain. I couldn't even take a sip of water without running to the toilet to hurl it back up again.

"Bex, I think you have alcohol poisoning," Jess said, when it was still happening at 4pm. "Should we go see a doctor?"

"Nope," I said, closing the door on her. I was tough, I

could take it. Meanwhile, my skull was pounding, and every breath I took caused my body to writhe in agony. Finally, hours later, I fell into a shallow, dreamless sleep that felt like a huge pool of relief.

I attempted to dial back my drinking, but the truth was, the more I damaged myself, the more I wanted to. While Jess began signing up for healthy activities like fun runs and water sports, I continued to party like there was no tomorrow.

~

There was just one problem with going out so much with colleagues. They were all there to witness your madness, and—even worse—to reflect it back to you in the cold light of Monday morning.

"I think I'm going to resign," I told Jess, on a particularly angst-ridden, hangover-filled morning.

"Really?" she asked. "Is the work that bad?"

It wasn't. The work was fine, but I was ashamed of my behaviour. I couldn't remember exactly what I'd done but I had vague recollections of making out with one of my colleagues in the middle of the dance floor. He was a sweet guy and I could tell by the way he looked at me that he liked me, so I felt even worse about it. What if he thought this was the start of something?

Worst of all, he was my supervisor.

Nope, best to find another job. At a new office, I could have a fresh start.

I didn't, though. I stayed there for another three years. The champagne functions were too good to pass up, and to be honest, I lacked the gumption to embark on a serious job-seeking mission. By day, I was a polite and cheerful creature. It was only at night that my inner wild child paraded around, dancing on tables, and waving her lunacy in the air.

In spite of my late-night penchant for self-destruction, I made a ton of party friendships. Most of the time I was bubbly and cheerful, and hell-bent on ensuring everyone had a great time. I was nominated for the office social committee, and attracted chuckles from management for the outrageous and fabulous ideas I came up with for our work events.

But deep down, I longed for more meaningful connections.

Often, I'd begin to form a real friendship with a girl from work, only to have to sheepishly text her the next morning, "Hey babe, do you know how I got home last night?"

More weekends than I could count were spent sick with anxiety over what I may have said or done, if only I could remember. On Monday mornings, I held my head up as best I could, meanwhile I died a little more inside. What the hell was wrong with me? Everyone loved Party Bex, until I'd inevitably take it too far. Nobody ever pulled me aside to tell me so, but I'd see concern in their eyes and it was all I could do to stop myself from running to the bathroom and crying. Why the hell couldn't I stop drinking when everyone else did?

By the end of each week, of course, all of this turmoil would be a distant memory and I'd be ready to paint the town red again, salivating in anticipation of that first delicious drink.

~

I met my second love in a crowded pub late one Friday night, after I'd lost Jess and left the dance floor to go searching for her. He asked me to dance, and then for my phone number, which I drunkenly keyed into his phone, closing one eye to help me focus. Then I promptly forgot all about it.

Seeing a call on my phone from an unknown number the following week, I let it go straight to voicemail. It was only when he left a message reminding me that we'd met on Friday night that I had a vague recollection of it. Not enough to remember anything about what he looked like, but enough to believe that it had, in fact, happened.

I was a little freaked out to realise that, even in that drunken state, I could remember my phone number and then have no memory of handing it out the next day. So I did what I always did. I ignored it. I deleted his message and pretended the whole thing never happened.

Only, he kept calling. A few days later, and again a few days after that. Finally, on a sunny Saturday afternoon two weeks after we'd first met, I answered. We chatted for ten minutes or so and he sounded nice enough, so when he asked me to meet him at the Bondi Hotel the following afternoon, I agreed. Bondi Hotel was large and pleasant, and close to my apartment. *If it's awful*, I reasoned, *I can always make a hasty exit.*

On the walk there, I felt nervous and more than a little foolish. It shouldn't have been a blind date, and yet, thanks to my crazy drinking, it was. I hadn't been brave enough to tell him that I had no clue what he looked like, so I hoped to God he recognised me before I spent ages scanning the pub like a mad woman.

As I pulled open the hotel door, I took a deep breath. *Here goes nothing.*

The bar was dimly lit, and it took a moment for my eyes to adjust. Just as the room came into focus, a man on a bar stool swivelled in my direction and leered. My stomach sank. *Oh God.* The look in his eyes made the hairs on the back of my neck stand up, and I was sorry I'd come. I knew I'd been drunk, but *holy shit.*

From the corner of my eye, I saw a blonde man approaching the door. Maybe I could just scurry out after him, and pretend this whole thing never happened.

"Hi Bex!" the blonde man smiled as he reached me. I turned to look at him and almost swooned with relief. This man's face looked sweet and kind, his manner gentle.

"I saved us a table through here," he said, leading me away from the main bar. The creepy guy swivelled his stool back to face the bar, and my heart attack subsided.

While Luke went to the bar, I texted Jess, "He's really nice. And cute!" Before I'd left home, I confided the whole sorry saga to her and naturally, she was worried.

"Haha, phew!" she messaged straight back, a second before he returned with our drinks.

Two years later, we were living together in his apartment overlooking Botany Bay. But we weren't happy. Drinking had turned out to be both our biggest common interest and our undoing. Unsure how to break the pattern we were in, I decided a fresh start was the answer.

On St Patricks Day, 2005, just a month shy of my thirtieth birthday, we boarded a one-way flight to Perth.

~

Back in Perth, I found work easily, despite being slightly hungover in the interview. I told the recruitment agency I wanted to move away from the banking industry. I wanted this move to signal a new beginning, and I blamed the banking industry for causing me to drink too much; all those functions just weren't good for me.

The agency placed me with a company in the oil and gas industry, complete with fabulous conditions and—wouldn't you know it—an entertainment budget that bordered on the obscene. I was worried for about five minutes, then I let myself get excited. It wouldn't be until many years later that they'd install breathalysers in the office, and conduct regular drug and alcohol screenings on their staff. 2005 was their heyday and I loved every minute of it.

The next eight years were a blur of champagne functions, dinners, weekend socialising, yachting, horse races, and disco bowling. Again, I made a ton of party friends, so there was always someone up for a laugh and a drink.

I was disappointed to find that the partying still came with a darker side. Losses of memory, handbags, jackets, dignity. Misunderstandings with friends. A twisted ankle that required thirteen weeks of physiotherapy to heal. *Not just the banking industry, then.* Luckily, I was well trained at focusing on the fun and ignoring anything else. Whenever I felt anxious about something I may have said or done, the solution came at 5pm in the form of a cheeky glass of sauvignon blanc.

Despite my drinking, I shone in annual work reviews. On one particularly hungover Monday in early 2011, my manager asked if I'd like to enrol to study a project management course at the company's expense. I jumped at the chance, delighted to have a reason to cut back on the socialising. I loved partying, but sometimes it all just felt so… *exhausting.* Often I found myself daydreaming about doing something more fulfilling with my life. Now I had my chance.

Six months later, after achieving one of the highest marks in the class despite my persistent hangovers, I was promoted to Cost Engineer.

~

"I need a hobby besides drinking!" I complained to my girlfriends over email every Monday morning as I nursed my coffee and pounding head.

In November 2011, quite by accident, I got my wish. After watching several traumatic documentaries about factory farming, I decided to follow a vegan lifestyle. I didn't know anyone who was vegan, and I received a ton of questions about what on earth I was going to eat. To keep myself accountable, and to share all the amazing concoctions (and spectacular fails) I was making in the kitchen, I started my first blog. Due to my penchant for glitter and excitable personality—especially after four glasses of sparkling wine—my friends and family often called me *Sparkles*. So I named the blog *Vegan Sparkles*.

I hadn't expected to fall in love with blogging. I thought I'd get bored with it after a month or two, like I always did with new interests. But in fact, it was just the opposite. My job was highly analytical, and I loved having a creative outlet. I also revelled in the support and energy of the vegan blogging community.

By the time The Institute for Integrative Nutrition in New York (also known as IIN) caught my attention in late 2012, my little blog had begun to grow a readership, and I'd started to feel a responsibility to be a healthy example of veganism, rather than an Oreo-crunching one. I discovered that many of the wellness bloggers I followed were graduates, and I was spellbound whenever I saw them with their green juices on Instagram.

"Are you stalking them again?" Dom laughed one day, catching me in the act.

"They're so inspiring," I giggled, looking up from my

phone. "Even on holidays, they're totally living the healthy lifestyle." It seemed a million miles away from my usual holiday folly of strong cocktails and late mornings.

"They are," Dom chuckled. "And soon it will be *you* inspiring others."

In a beautiful flash of synchronicity, I also heard about an online business and marketing program called B-School. It reminded me of a documentary my friend, Sophie, and I had seen years earlier. In the film, they suggested that certain people were predisposed to entrepreneurship; they were just wired for the excitement of it. On the flip side, they were also predisposed to addiction.

"So *that's* my problem," I'd laughed. "I just need to become an entrepreneur!" It was a wisecrack designed to take the sting out of being so hungover that day, but what if it were true? I certainly didn't see myself as an entrepreneur, but I became enchanted with the idea of it.

After much deliberation, I took the plunge and enrolled in both courses. For months, my life was a cycle of work, study, sleep, rinse, repeat. But far from feeling drained, a strange thing began to happen. I started to feel energised, inspired, and *alive*.

# THREE

My phone buzzed with a new message from Dom, "DONE! My boss accepted my resignation with regret, but wished me well in our venture. Exciting!" Dom worked in the technology industry, but wanted to start his own graphic design and web development business, as well as help me with my website.

I texted him back, "Oh wow, it's happening! I'm still shaking! So exciting!"

Still grinning like a lunatic, I came up with my next fabulous idea. I decided to host an event to celebrate our business launch, with Dom helping behind the scenes. I'd recently been to a fun wellness event hosted by a health coach, and it didn't seem all that difficult to organise. I figured it'd be a great way to get the word out, plus it would give me something concrete to focus on, to keep the nerves at bay. Since I was required to give four weeks notice, I decided to host the event the day after my last day at work.

"You're amazing," Jenna shook her head in disbelief and admiration when I finally found her and told her about my event ideas. Jenna was a close friend in my current team, and I'd miss her most of all. We'd been going for coffee dates in our building's lobby café for months now and it was the only part of the morning I looked forward to.

"Well, if we're gonna' do this, we've gotta' be *all in*, baby! We've gotta' hustle!" I joked, and we fell about laughing. I was scared, but I also felt pure excitement. It was the same feeling I used to get at 5pm every Friday, before we all headed out for drinks. Like anything could happen. And if I could feel this way without all of the chaos that alcohol got me into, well, things were looking very rosy indeed.

The next few weeks were a blur of accountant and legal appointments, opening business bank accounts, viewing potential event venues, booking yoga teachers, sourcing superfood ingredients, and researching ticketing options. We also got busy updating our websites and revising our LinkedIn profiles, hoping someone might know someone who might be our perfect client.

On my final day of work, I couldn't stop looking at the clock. Why did six hours in a bar feel like six minutes, while eight hours before the start of your new life felt like eight million of the most gruelling hours on earth?

Just when I decided I couldn't take the torture any longer and packed up my bag to leave, Jenna called out from Sean's office, "Hey hon, can you come in here for a sec?"

I put my bag down and went to see how I could help. There, crowded in Sean's office, were my team mates with a huge bunch of flowers and a giant card. As they wished me well, I couldn't help getting emotional. *I was going to miss these guys.*

After hugging them all farewell, I skipped all the way home. This felt like the fresh start I so desperately needed.

~

Six days later, Rosie flew into Perth from Sydney. Rosie and I had formed a close friendship years ago, while working on the reception desk of a recruitment agency, just before I moved to London. I hadn't seen her in months and I'd been counting down the days until she arrived.

We met at a fancy waterfront bar near the city. It was a beautiful spring day and I was thrilled to see her. All dolled up in our favourite frocks, we hugged and squealed hello.

"I'll get the first bottle," I said. "Go pick a table you like."

When I returned with a champagne bottle and two flutes, I found her waving her menu at me from an outdoor table. "This one!" she giggled, gesturing towards the view. Sunshine sparkled across the water. It was perfect.

"I can't *believe* you both resigned," she said, folding her menu away. "Give me the goss, girlfriend!"

I told her about the wellness event I'd hosted the day after we finished work. How much fun it was, and how I'd stayed sober the night before, even though it was a Friday!

"And I was clever, you see," I grinned. "I scheduled my farewell party in my second-last week of work, so I was nicely recovered before my wellness event."

"I'm so proud of you!" she smiled. I scanned her face. If she noticed how mixed up my logic was, she didn't let on. An icky feeling had come over me. Like I was a fraud, glugging back booze while simultaneously telling her about my health coaching practice, but I shrugged it off. I'd been so good since I left the corporate world. *I deserved this.*

Over our second bottle, she told me all about her up-coming travel and renovation plans, and showed me a bunch of photos on her phone.

By 5pm, we'd already polished off three bottles and were drunkenly contemplating a fourth. Rosie's husband Peter arrived fresh from work, and the look on his face made it blatantly clear that he was aghast at the state of us.

He pulled a chair up to our table and sat down. And then the curtain falls. That's the last thing I remember.

~

The next morning, while I tried not to cry, Dom filled me in on the missing details. With a deep sigh, he described how I'd staggered through the front door, straight past him, and promptly passed out, face-down, on the couch.

In my hand was a paper bag. And inside that paper bag was an unopened bottle of wine.

"I've never seen you like that before," he said, staring into my soul. "This took it up a notch. Seriously. You scared me."

Which in turn, scared *me*. How the hell had I managed to get another bottle? Was it from the waterfront bar?

I was terrified to text Rosie, worried about the state I'd been in when she bid me farewell. Was she mad at me? Did she put me into a taxi? Did Peter think I was a bad influence? I felt sick not knowing.

With a shaky hand, I texted her, "It was so good to see you yesterday, honey!" I clicked 'send', and held my breath. When she didn't text back immediately, I tried to convince myself she was busy getting brunch or something, and not just ignoring me. I slipped my phone into the bottom of my bag to stop myself from checking it every other minute, but it was no use. I was wallowing in my pool of misery now, letting my fingers get all wrinkly in it.

An eternity passed. Finally, she texted back, "God, I'm so hungover! I love you so much!"

I almost cried with relief. I wanted to call her and ask her how I got home, but I was too ashamed. Better to just hope it all ended fairly well, and move on. As I put my phone away, I still felt sick.

I was an idiot and an imposter; this was less than a week after my *wellness* event. I had one foot in my new lifestyle and one firmly stuck in the old one, and I couldn't figure out how on earth to reconcile them. What if one of my clients had seen me being poured into a taxi? What kind of message was I sending them? Not to mention that this kind of behaviour was not appropriate for a woman my age, especially one who proclaimed the virtues of holistic health. *Good grief.*

A couple of days later, I was walking past my local bottle store when my heart skipped a beat. It wasn't so much a flashback as a blinding flash of just 'knowing' that was where I'd bought the mystery bottle of wine. What sort of incoherent mess was I in by then? What did the guy behind the counter think? I shuddered and vowed to drink more water next time, and to stay away from champagne during the day. *How many times did I need to learn this lesson?*

One thing was for damn sure; I wouldn't be heading back to that particular bottle store any time soon.

~

Three months later I awoke to a familiar intensity that felt suspiciously like a hideous hangover.

*What? No, it can't be! I must be dreaming,* I told myself sleepily. I stumbled to the shower, desperate for the hot water to wash away this sense of dread and give me clarity.

Flashbacks of the night danced before my eyes. Excited by the first chance to enjoy our large rooftop area in the warmer weather, we invited a dozen friends over for an outdoor movie night. Louise brought a projector, we set up our stereo speakers, and everyone brought cushions and bean bags to sit on. We met in our apartment first to get the snacks and drinks all organised. I made popcorn and mini pastries, and loved catching up with everyone. I topped up drinks and was the perfect hostess. *One drink for you, one drink for me.*

By the time we settled in to watch the movie, I felt quite drunk, and not really in the mood to settle down for a movie at all. I wanted to party! As the movie's theme song played behind the intro credits, I sang along, dancing in my chair.

And then what? I scanned my brain's databank. *Error: file not found.*

*No!* I stomped my feet in the shower. This couldn't be happening again. For three months, I'd controlled my drinking. I still always wanted more, but I managed to stop after two or three glasses, and felt proud as punch of my progress. *That incident with Rosie was clearly just a left-over from my corporate mindset*, I told myself. *Things were going to be different around here.*

Dom and I had even been on a trip to Sydney, and I managed to hold it together. We hosted another wellness event, and despite my nerves, I kept a lid on it. We went to Rosie's fortieth birthday party, and I did an incredible impression of drinking like a lady. Throughout the whole trip, I still had cocktails and wine every night, of course— it was a *holiday*—but I didn't go overboard like I had on every other holiday I'd ever been on. At long last, *progress.*

Only, it seemed it wasn't progress. Just false hope.

When I finally got out of the shower, I apologised to

Dom.

"Maybe you should drive today," he suggested, knowing that I was heading to Cara's baby shower that afternoon, at a fancy hotel complete with high tea and champagne. For a split second, I contemplated it, but the idea seemed preposterous. I mean, who doesn't drink at a baby shower, besides the Mums-to-be?

"I won't drink too much, I'm already hungover," I mumbled, tears welling in my eyes.

He dropped me off at the front of the hotel. It was gorgeous, with ornate brass railings and marble floors surrounding a large indoor fountain. There were about a dozen of us, dressed up in our party frocks, looking every bit the sophisticated ladies. I attempted to eat canapés and sip champagne, but I was still feeling too wretched to really enjoy them. The ladies chatted as they helped themselves to the buffet. I knew about half of the guests, and it was fun to mingle with them.

Eventually I found myself seated with Louise and Meghan, both of whom had been at our movie night. My eyes scanned their body language and faces for telltale signs of a hangover, but they didn't seem to be afflicted at all.

"You're not eating much," Louise nodded towards my empty plate, before taking a bite of a mini sandwich. "Were there not many vegan choices up there?"

"No, no. There were. I'm just suffering a bit after last night. And Dom's mad at me," I confided.

"Huh? For what?" she asked, taking a sip of her champagne.

"For being too drunk and rowdy last night." I didn't have to bring it up, but I wanted her to tell me that Dom was overreacting and that I hadn't been as drunk as I imagined. In my paranoid, anxious state, I desperately needed reassurance that everything was going to be fine. That *I* was going to be fine.

"Oh, what? You weren't! You were *fine*, babe. We were *all* a bit merry," Louise said, ever the loyal friend. I wasn't sure I believed her this time, any more than I'd believed her the hundreds of times before, but I loved her for saying it all the same.

Meghan looked at me and then looked away, before changing the subject. I got the distinct impression that she agreed with Dom, and for a second I felt mad at her for not coming to my defence.

My anger quickly turned to shame. I thought about how Meghan acted in front of her man; always so graceful and respectable. I didn't want to be the brash, loud-mouthed lush—I wanted to be graceful and respectable too. I felt like crying, but instead I sipped my champagne and tried to put on a brave face. *I'm just hungover, that's all,* I reasoned. *This afternoon I'll arrive home like a lady, and this will all feel better tomorrow.*

Three days later, Rosie was flying into Perth again and I was to meet her, and two of our girlfriends, for a ladies lunch complete with champagne. I'd prove it to Dom then. I'd be so well behaved, his head would spin!

And three days later, I tried. I really did. But somewhere around the fourth glass of champagne, all my good intentions went out the window. The only thing that mattered was coveting the next drink.

~

Evidently, I needed more rules. I was about to start my first online group coaching program. I *had* to get a handle on this thing.

On the first Monday in 2014, I launched *The Sparkle Project*, teaching nourishment of body, mind and soul. I spent weeks creating the content, while Dom designed the web pages, emails, and program workbooks. With thirty-six coaching sessions booked into my calendar over six weeks, I knew my schedule would be demanding, but I was excited about obtaining more coaching practice and checking in with our members.

To steady my nerves, I leaned on my old friend, wine. But with strict rules this time. A single bottle of wine on Friday nights, followed by a single bottle on Saturday nights, followed by five days alcohol-free. It was a tough regimen, but I was sticking to it. *So far, so good.*

I remembered a work team-building event I'd been to years before, when one of my colleagues had refused a drink. "I only allow myself to drink on Wednesdays, Fridays, and Sundays," she confided. "Otherwise, where does it end?" I nodded, bemused. I'd made many rules about my drinking over the years, like 'I'm only drinking cider, not wine', 'I'm having two alcohol-free days per week' and 'I'm only having four drinks', with varying levels of failure.

There were no real repercussions for breaking those rules. It could all be laughed off with a jolly 'Oops! Better luck next week.'

But it didn't feel so hilarious anymore. It felt hard to stick to, and that worried me. I hated the version of me that pitched a fit if Dom tried to pour himself a glass from one of my precious, single bottles. I hated that I felt anxious as I neared the end of the bottle, especially on Saturday nights, when I knew the next scheduled drink was so very far away.

Our local bottle store was still off-limits, obviously, since I wasn't sure if I'd made a complete fool of myself after that boozy waterfront lunch with Rosie four months prior. Instead, I started driving to a new bottle store in the suburbs. It was a large discount warehouse kind of place, and they often had specials on wine when you bought a half-dozen at once. Each time I bought one of those special packs, I promised myself I'd make it last three weeks. But somehow I found myself driving back there every week. Friends didn't only visit on the weekends, plus there were midweek colleague catch-ups, movie nights, and birthdays. And once I'd bent my strict rule a few times, it seemed perfectly acceptable to crack open a new bottle mid-week after a particularly stressful day, or whenever we had something to celebrate.

Sometimes I'd find myself standing in front of an empty fridge on a Friday afternoon. *Oops. How did that happen?*

"I'll go get us some groceries," I chirped to Dom, tell-

ing myself that was most definitely all I was going out for.
Sometimes I'd make it back home with just the groceries.
More often than not, my brain turned into a bloody bat-
tlefield for the entire trip.

*Okay, I won't buy wine tonight because I want to feel bet-
ter.*

*But what if someone comes over and I don't have anything
in the house for them?*

*If I don't drink tonight, I'll get up early tomorrow and go
to the farmers market and feel all happy and healthy.*

*But it's Friday! It's normal to let loose on Friday, I've
worked so hard all week!*

*If I get a bottle, I'll only fall asleep with my face in my
glass in front of the TV later tonight.*

*So? Live a little! Don't be so boring!*

On and on the battle would rage. So much energy and
headspace wasted, going back and forth. Whichever side
won, by the time I got home I was cranky and exhausted.
Either win felt like a hollow, temporary victory.

The battle may have been over, but the war had only
just begun.

~

Later that month, to celebrate Australia Day, we were invited to a party at Chloé's. We hadn't seen much of our
friends since launching our own business. Chloé's apartment had a large balcony overlooking the city, guarantee-
ing a fabulous view of the evening fireworks.

Dom and I arrived late in the afternoon. I was stressed out and overwhelmed by the huge amount of work waiting for us at home. I also had a bee in my bonnet about something a friend had said to me the day before, and grumpy that we'd arrived after everyone else already had a buzz on.

We'd brought three bottles of wine with us, because I always got antsy if we only had two. *What if someone else wanted a glass? What if we ran out halfway through the party and all the bottle stores were closed?* Dom wasn't happy about this, but I convinced him it was a good idea 'just in case' and that I would take it easy and not go too crazy— *promise!* I was skating on very thin ice where my drinking was concerned, and I knew it.

It was the perfect storm. Tired, stressed, overwhelmed, upset about some perceived—ridiculous—slight, and at a party for the first time in ages with a huge group of friends. Naturally, I drank like a sailor, determined to have *the best time ever!* I flirted like mad, danced like a woman possessed, lost my shoes, yelled inappropriate things across the room, and got so completely sloppy drunk that I didn't remember the ride home.

~

The next morning, as I'd done a thousand times, I woke up desperately trying to piece together the night before. *Where were my shoes? Did I lose my handbag? Was Dom mad at me?*

I opened one eye and saw that he wasn't in bed next to

me. The bedroom door was closed. My stomach lurched. *Oh God.*

I climbed out of bed as gingerly as possible, and made a beeline for the ensuite shower. Maybe if I pretended I wasn't hungover, the whole night would be forgotten. Maybe there was nothing for him to be mad about anyway. Maybe the point where my memory shatters is just the point where I fell asleep, and I'm worrying for nothing. *That's possible, right?*

In the shower, I felt desperately alone. My emotions see-sawed from righteous indignation—*for God's sake, what's the big deal, everyone binge drinks!*—to feeling completely lost and unloveable.

As I dressed, I tried not to cry. Taking a deep and shaky breath, I opened the bedroom door as softly as I could and headed to the kitchen to retrieve a glass of water.

"And how are *you* feeling this morning?" Dom asked loudly, sneaking up behind me and scaring the living daylights out of me.

"Okay," I mumbled, still gauging the situation. My blurry eyes betrayed me and I couldn't read him.

"Oh, *really?*" he pressed.

"Really!" I surprised myself by yelling. He could wipe that smug look off his face. He knew that I was dying to know what had happened, and yet, he was going to make me suffer. Because he knew damn well that not knowing was the worst.

He walked away, knowing better than to get into a tangle with a madwoman.

*I'd show him just how fine I was, I fumed. I'd fix my hair and put on make-up, and maybe even go out somewhere for the day, and not tell him where I was going. See how he liked being kept in the dark.*

While I attempted to apply mascara with shaky hands, he tried again. "I would have thought you'd be feeling rather rough indeed…"

"I'm FINE!" I hollered.

"I don't think you are," he said, staring me down.

My face flushed with the heat of a thousand suns. Why was it so hot in here all of a sudden? I needed space, and privacy, dammit. Couldn't he see I was doing *womanly things?*

"*Everybody* drinks," I declared.

"No, they don't. Not like that." His gaze remained even and it infuriated the hell out of me.

Everyone I knew *did* binge drink at some point. Why did *I* have a problem, and not them?

"Well, if only we could all be as perfect as *you* and your family!" I shouted, slamming the bathroom door in his face.

I didn't even know what that meant.

*But how dare he judge me! I didn't have to take this crap. Maybe I should just break up with him, then I could do whatever the hell I wanted. I could drink any damn time I liked. If I didn't care how I was treating myself, why should he care?*

Only, I did care. It just frightened me to admit it.

I caught my reflection in the mirror. *Seriously?* A small part of me whispered, *You're about to choose your love of drinking over the love you've dreamt of your entire life?*

I started to cry.

What was I doing? What person in their right mind would choose alcohol over their soul mate?

A wave of shame and nausea washed over me, threatening to drown me completely.

In desperation, I swung the door open and ran to him, almost breaking the door handle in the process. I was sobbing so hard, I thought I might throw up. "I'm sorry! I don't know what's wrong with me. What's wrong with me?"

# FOUR

Two weeks later, Sophie and her husband John invited us over for a housewarming dinner. Sophie and I had been best friends since high school. She moved to Brisbane when we were in our early twenties. We'd visited each other, of course, and spent hours on the phone, but I was so excited that she'd finally moved back to Perth.

"Now, take it easy tonight," Dom warned me on the drive over.

"I will!" I sang, with a cheeky smile.

We went to Meghan's engagement party the weekend before. The guests included the same circle of friends that were at Chloé's party, and I was determined to prove that

I could just have a few drinks and not get messy. "I was good last week, wasn't I?" I couldn't resist asking Dom.

"You almost had too much—," he began.

"But I didn't."

"Well, you were a bit silly on the way home…" he trailed off, as he pulled the car into Sophie's driveway.

My recollection of the trip home from the engagement party was a little fuzzy, but the fact that he couldn't name any humiliation in particular felt like a huge triumph. *Yes! In your* face, *drinking-too-much!* This was it. *Finally*. After decades of trying—and failing—to moderate my drinking, I was going to be the mature, sophisticated drinker I so longed to be.

As always, I had a dilemma deciding how many bottles of wine to bring that night. Dom had offered to drive, so he wouldn't have more than a glass or two, but how many would I need? I thought about Chloé's party for the millionth time, and fought my urge to pack three bottles. Two would do it. Better to be safe than sorry. I had new skills to show off, right? Besides, Sophie and her hubby loved wine too, so I was fairly certain they'd have plenty of back-up bottles. You know, just in case.

Dinner was delicious. John made wood-fired pizzas, and the smell was amazing on the balmy summer air. We sat around the large wooden table on their back verandah, laughing over their moving mishap stories. I drank slowly and steadily and felt very in control.

"Shall we make a move?" Dom asked me at about 10pm.

"Just one more?" I replied, reaching for the bottle to refill my glass. I watched him to see if he seemed shitty. I didn't want to push my luck so soon after our big argument, but he didn't seem concerned.

Soon enough, I finished that glass too. I knew it was time to call it a night but I didn't want to stop drinking. I never did. The buzz was too good. I quickly considered my options. I didn't want to make Dom stay longer than he wanted to, and I didn't want to argue in front of our hosts. *Could I have another couple of glasses at home, maybe?* Dom had tolerated my couch drinking in the past, but I wasn't sure if he'd put up with it now. Not after Chloé's party.

When would I be able to drink again? I scanned the upcoming week in my mind. I'd been invited to a girls night out with ex-colleagues on Tuesday night. That was only three nights away. Valentines Day was just three days after that, and everyone knew that champagne was mandatory on Valentines Day.

"Okay, let's go, mister," I said, rising from the table, feeling like a poster child for moderation. *Look at me go!* This was a new me; all mature, wonderful, and lady-like.

～

Tuesday morning, on my way to lunch, Jenna sent me a text message. "Unfortunately everyone seems to be a bit busy just now and the ladies can't manage tonight. Rescheduled for a lunch date on Thursday next week if you can manage then, chica?"

I checked my calendar, and wrote back to let her know I'd be there.

Oh well, I'd save money by not heading into the city that night. Plus, I had lunch plans to look forward to.

I was meeting my gorgeous health coach friends, Holly and Zara, at a funky new health café just north of the city. As I walked in, I spotted Holly already seated at a cosy table in the corner.

"Hi gorgeous!" she cooed, as we hugged hello.

Zara arrived a moment later and we both hugged her.

"This place is so beautiful," Zara said, admiring our surroundings. Sunshine streamed through the large windows, and bare brick walls showcased fun pop art.

Just then, a new group arrived and settled into a larger table towards the back. Some of their faces looked strangely familiar. I couldn't help staring, racking my brain to figure out where I knew them from. Suddenly, it clicked. There were eight people in the party, and I recognised at least three of them as superstars in the wellness world.

"Oh my God, it's Jo and Mia," Holly whispered, clearly recognising them at the same time. As I looked at her, I knew we both felt too awkward to go up and say hi.

"This is so weird," Holly giggled. "Jacqueline actually emailed me this morning, asking if I knew of anyone who could volunteer at their event tonight, because they're one short. I haven't actually met Jacqueline, but I'm pretty sure that's her at their table as well."

"Well, what about you, Bex?" Zara asked. "Can you come?"

"Oh," I said, completely caught off guard. I vaguely remembered hearing about this upcoming event, but I'd been working too hard to really take notice. "Tonight? Where is it?"

"It's at the Empyrean Centre in Northbridge," Holly jumped in, grinning her approval of the idea. "The volunteers are called 'Earth Angels' and we get to watch the event for free as a thank you for helping out. We're both going, and so are Kristy and Carly. It'll be fun!"

"Okay," I laughed. Now that my girls night out had been postponed, my night was free, and it might be fun to have a spontaneous adventure. "What do I need to do?"

"Just wear all-black and be there at 4pm," Zara said, taking a sip of her berry smoothie.

"I guess we'll officially meet them then," Holly said, nodding towards the large table at the back.

⁓

After lunch, I drove home and went through my wardrobe. *All black? Hmm.* Over the past few months, I'd traded most of my black corporate wear for more bright and colourful hues. Finally, at the back of my wardrobe, I found a black skirt and shirt.

"I'll drop you off," Dom offered. He was the *real* Earth Angel.

I hadn't been to that particular theatre before. It was gorgeous inside, with plush, richly coloured carpet and elegant fittings. I found Holly, Zara, and Kristy sitting together in the lobby, and quickly joined them.

"Bex, this is Erin," Kristy said, gesturing to a pretty blonde girl to her right.

"Wait. Are you Vegan Sparkles?" Erin asked, her eyes widening.

I chuckled, nodding. "I'm Bex. Nice to meet you."

"*Wow*, this night is blowing my mind already!" she said, and we all laughed.

Suddenly, I felt relieved that I hadn't had a drink in three days. My wellness world and my drinking world were becoming harder and harder to reconcile.

"Welcome, ladies!" a woman said loudly, as she joined the group. "I'm Jacqueline. Thank you so much for helping out tonight, we're so happy to have you. If you'd like to follow me, we'll head upstairs where we'll divvy up the duties."

We grabbed our things and followed her lead. Upstairs, another small group of volunteers waited to be assigned. Holly, Erin, and I were nominated to man the front doors as the audience members arrived. Jacqueline handed us each an iPad and talked us through how to check off names as guests presented their tickets. Fully briefed, we headed downstairs to assume our positions.

"I wonder if we should tell them that they won't be doing much business tonight?" Holly joked as she nodded towards the bar that lined the entire back wall of the foyer. Two bar staff waited eagerly for the venue doors to swing open.

"Yeah," I let out a small laugh. I knew what she meant;

this was a wellness crowd, not your regular theatre goers. I thought about all the evening events I'd ever been to, and how cranky I would have been if there'd been no alcohol available. Art gallery exhibitions, speaking events, live gigs, theatre; they were all accompanied by the obligatory glass of wine or three. If I'd paid to come to this event, would I have bought a glass of wine? *Pretty damn likely*. Surely, Holly was a little mistaken, and other people would buy drinks too?

A side door opened and Jo and Mia walked in, looking every bit the wellness goddesses they were. Their long, shiny curls bounced around the shoulders of their flowing gowns. Their faces glowed with health and happiness.

"Hi guys!" they waved and smiled at us, as they made their way upstairs.

"Hi!" we waved back, a little starstruck.

This was a huge night for them. They were about to go on stage and speak to an audience of hundreds, and you can bet your bottom dollar they wouldn't be sipping champagne in the green room. Green *juice* room, more like it.

Theatre staff swung open the main doors, interrupting my train of thought. Outside, a small queue had already formed. Holly, Erin and I got busy, matching names and checking guests in.

For the next hour, I kept one eye on the task at hand at the other firmly on the bar.

I'd been to another evening event recently when one of my favourite IIN lecturers, David Wolfe, came to town. Dom accompanied me, and we met up with a couple of my health coach friends. I didn't have a drink that night, but there was no temptation to, either. That venue didn't have a bar.

This event was different entirely. I couldn't help but watch with fascination that bordered on obsession. So far, only a dozen people out of a hundred or so had approached the bar. *Twelve percent!* Wow. I wondered what my corporate friends would make of an event like this.

On and on, people streamed into the foyer, and I continued to clock the bar. Any minute now, the pre-show bells would chime and they'd miss their chance to buy a drink. Didn't they *know* that?

Sure enough, *bing bing bing.* Theatre staff removed the velvet ropes and ushered everyone upstairs. I watched the bar, expecting a mad, last-minute dash that never came. *Huh.* These people really were just here for the talk. I wondered if they were waiting to get one at intermission, but somehow I doubted it.

"Okay ladies, follow me," Jacqueline appeared again, motioning for us to follow her upstairs. In the upstairs foyer, we saw that all the guests had disappeared into the theatre and the other volunteers were gathered in a group, waiting for us. Another woman ran up, handing us each a bottle of green juice.

"Once the event begins, I'll lead you to a section where you can watch the show," Jacqueline instructed. "We'll meet here again afterwards."

We popped the tops off our juices and nodded. A few minutes later, we silently followed Jacqueline to the back of the theatre.

"Along here," she whispered, gesturing to the section behind the sound and lighting guys. From our standing position, we had a great view, and I was excited to see these guys talk. I hadn't been to a wellness event this large before.

A well-known singer-songwriter kicked off the show with a magical solo. Goosebumps tingled along my spine. I was so grateful to be there.

Finally, Jo walked on stage. It was her event, organised to celebrate her recent book launch. She was a tiny little thing, so petite, and yet she commanded every inch of the stage. Her voice was full of confidence and conviction as she shared her story of cancer that had threatened her young life. I watched in awe. She was a decade younger than me and yet she was doing so much in the world, and with her life in general.

Next, Jo invited three guests onto the stage—the singer-songwriter, a guy I didn't recognise, and Mia—and introduced them all as her close friends. They sat in large armchairs lined along the stage, and began to talk about their journeys into living a healthy life. The other guy was also a musician and, in fact, the owner of the café we'd all had lunch in earlier that day. The conversation was casual, and even awkward at times. I decided to sit on the carpet and just listen. A few of the other volunteers followed suit, no doubt feeling a little pooped after our duties, and likely having skipped dinner too.

To my surprise, the conversation on stage moved to alcohol. In particular, how to handle being sober in a huge drinking culture. *Well, this was unexpected.* Fascinated, I hung on their every word. What *was* it like to be sober in Australia? I didn't know *anyone* who didn't drink. What made them decide they'd never drink again, and how did they handle it?

The two guys talked about how challenging it had been at first, and how some of their old friends still didn't understand it. They each had health issues that were better managed by remaining sober, and yet people still pressured them to drink. Jo chimed in, agreeing that it was marginally easier to 'get away with' sobriety when you had a life-threatening illness. She expressed sympathy for anyone who wanted to stop drinking just because they wanted to be healthier. They all laughed about meditation being their new 'high', and I made a mental note to try it with more enthusiasm.

As they talked, I thought about the strange series of events that had led me here; to this theatre, in this very moment, so soon after the incident at Chloé's party. My ex-colleagues postponing our girls night out, the event organisers being a volunteer short, having a lunch date with Holly and Zara that day who, unbeknownst to me, had signed up as volunteers. It didn't feel like a coincidence. It felt like I was meant to be right here, sitting cross-legged on the floor, absorbing every word.

Just before the talk finished, Jacqueline appeared again, and silently motioned for us to follow. Back in the upstairs foyer, she nominated Holly, Erin and I to help facilitate the meet-and-greet. I was asked to follow the sing-er-songwriter with a collection of pens and notepaper so he could easily sign autographs for guests.

As I followed this talented man around, I marvelled at the stories people came up to confide in him. They de-scribed the myriad of ways his songs and his message had changed their lives for the better. Even more beautiful was his humble, caring nature as he listened to every word.

None of the people involved in this event seemed to be worried about where their next drink was coming from. They weren't counting down the minutes until they could cut loose with a bottle of bubbles. They were devoted to growth, to sharing their message, and making an impact. Most of all, they were completely present and conscious in every moment of their own lives.

I realised that, more than anything in the world, I wanted that too.

~

I wish I could say that I stopped drinking that night. Or three nights later, on Valentines Day, when I found my-self hiding an empty wine bottle from Dom. We'd bought a single bottle to share, but craving a refill without an ar-gument, I topped up my glass from a bottle at the back of the fridge when he wasn't looking. It was only when I woke the next morning that I remembered the empty bot-tle in the back of the cupboard. *Oh God, what if he found it?* We'd had plenty of arguments about my drinking, but I was sure that they were *nothing* compared to the battle that would ensue if he found that bottle.

In the shower, I racked my brain, wondering what the hell to do with it. If I put it in the recycling box, he'd see it and ask why it wasn't there the night before. Could I hide it somewhere else? Maybe I could run it down to the outside bin while he was in the shower, and he'd be none the wiser?

When he finally left to visit his brother, I ran with it, hungover and paranoid, down to the bin. As I rode back up in the elevator, I felt a new level of shame. All this sneaking around, it felt awful. Even if he didn't catch me, I was sure he could sense it, and that I was voluntarily damaging our relationship.

I didn't like where this was heading.

A week or so later, one of my beautiful clients confided that she drank to make herself feel less lonely. To my sheer horror, I heard myself say, "That's okay." I felt sick the second the words left my lips, because I knew in my heart that it wasn't okay. That it was never okay to use alcohol— or food, or drugs—to numb ourselves or avoid what was really going on in our lives. I felt disgusted with myself. I owed my clients more than that, and most of all, I owed it to myself. In that moment, I vowed to be a better example, and to sort this mess out once and for all.

But I didn't stop. Each event stayed with me, haunting me in the back of my mind, whispering to me.

A month after the Earth Angels event, on a balmy Saturday night in March, Louise hosted a party for our group of friends. Her long-awaited courtyard renovations were finally finished, and what better excuse to celebrate?

I was so excited to catch up with the whole gang. I was *fairly* sure I hadn't said or done anything stupid at Meghan's engagement party the month before. Plus, I figured the more times they saw me as 'Party Bex', the faster they'd forget 'Sloppy Drunk Bex' they'd witnessed at Chloé's.

In the past, I'd always had a glass of champagne—or two, or three—while I got ready, just to get into the festive mood. But this time I was extra cautious. I had two bottles of wine packed, and I was skipping the pre-drinks altogether. As I looked in the mirror, I gave myself a nod of approval. *See? I can be an adult. I will learn to moderate or die trying.*

"Cab's here!" Dom called. I gathered my bag and jacket and walked out the door with a spring in my step.

~

"Bex!" Louise exclaimed when we arrived, pulling me into a hug. "Here, have a glass of this, it's so yummy," she said, handing me a glass of sparkling rosé. I took a sip.

"Ooooh, it's lovely!" I cooed. I thought about the two bottles of wine in our cooler bag, and my self-imposed limit. Oh well, I could always share those bottles with everyone later. I still planned to only drink one bottle myself in total. Maybe one and a half. But no more. *Absolutely* no more than that.

"Come on, come and see it all!" Louise said, ushering me into the courtyard.

Dom was out there, chatting to the guys with a glass of wine in his hand. I wasn't sure if it was from one of our bottles, but if it was, I hoped to hell he was drinking it slowly.

*See?* If we'd just brought three bottles like usual, I wouldn't even be *having* these thoughts. I hated this! What if we ran out?

Another friend arrived and I snapped out of it. I noticed that she'd brought two bottles of wine with her. I quickly scanned the courtyard to see how many other bottles were waiting nearby. A lot, it seemed. Okay, maybe we'd be safe after all.

Brooke and Mark arrived next, and Brooke asked if I'd like to try a glass of sparkling wine they'd bought from their trip to the vineyards down south. "Ooh, yes please," I nodded, secretly worried that my rations of wine would be gone by now. Dom rarely drank more than three glasses, but who knows! Anything could happen. Anyway, I liked these bubbles better than the wines we'd brought. They were more festive. I'd share whatever was left of our bottles later.

Soon enough, another bottle of bubbles was passed around and my glass was topped up. My counting got a little fuzzy. Was it three glasses I'd had, or four? I figured I should probably switch to my own wine. These bubbles were disorienting me.

I went into Louise's kitchen to search for the largest

wine glass I could find. On my way back outside, I ran into Louise giving Meghan a tour of her bedroom and hallway renovations.

"Oh my goodness, we watched the funniest thing today," I said, grabbing Louise's arm. I launched into a rambling description of a scene from a television show, and cracked myself up laughing. Louise and Meghan giggled but seemed a little confused by my story, so I decided to go outside and tell it again. See if I got a better reaction this time. Maybe I needed to put more emphasis on the punch line.

I poured myself a wine, and tried again. Still not the reaction I was hoping for.

*Jeepers,* everyone was a bit dull tonight. Didn't they know this was a *party?* I poured myself yet another glass, and walked over to another couple of friends. They seemed the least amused of the bunch.

*Oh well, I'd just amuse myself then!* I thought of a few other funny stories in my head and laughed out loud, but couldn't be bothered to share them. No-one seemed to appreciate my humour tonight anyway. I quickly got bored and poured myself another glass.

And that's where my memory calls it a night.

~

What felt like five minutes later, I slowly opened my eyes. I could already tell it was going to hurt. A jackhammer had taken up residence in my skull and my body ached.

Oh, how it ached.

*No, no, NO!* I silently screamed in frustration. *Not again!*

I dragged myself into the ensuite shower, moving as quietly as possible so I wouldn't wake Dom. I couldn't bear an argument right now.

After showering, I felt marginally better, but for the most part, like death warmed up. I took my time brushing my teeth, nervous about facing Dom. When I finally came out of the bathroom, he was already in the living room. And just as I'd suspected, he was grumpy. But there was a new emotion mixed in there as well. Something like resignation. Defeat.

"You were messy last night," he said, with a slight crack in his voice. There was sadness in his eyes and my heart broke a little more, knowing I was the cause.

"Everyone else was drunk too!" I said, my cheeks burning.

"No. Everyone else has grown up a bit," he replied.

*Well, where was my memo on* that? I wondered. *When did everyone else decide to become all mature and sensible, leaving me to carry on the party alone?*

I sat on the couch in a huff, mulling it all over. Come to think of it, I couldn't remember the last time I'd seen any of our friends get drunker than me. It used to happen sometimes when we'd be out every Friday night, but not often. I usually wore the drunkest crown. Actually, no-one had contested the throne for quite some time.

*Oh my God, was I the lush of the group?* I thought about

a woman I knew through another group of friends. I partied a lot with that group when I was in my early thirties
and she was in her early fifties. She was always messy, even
at the very start of the night, waving her wine glass around
and telling stories with glassy eyes. Everyone avoided her
like the plague towards the end of the night, because if
you weren't careful, she'd latch on to your arm and yell
the same story over and over, before finally—thankfully—
slumping into a nearby chair. I remember thinking, *Good*
grief*, I hope I don't turn out like her.*

There was another woman in that group of friends who
was pretty wild too. I was on holiday with my family in
Bali, when she met us, and a few other friends, for sunset
drinks at a beachside bar.

"Vodka! I brought my own," she said as she arrived,
slamming her water bottle down on the table. I was a huge
drinker, but even *my* eyes widened in surprise. Straight
vodka from a water bottle. *Wow.* She drank the entire
thing, too, and proceeded to fall apart in front of our eyes.

After sunset, we all walked down to a nearby Chinese
restaurant. She got rowdy, grabbing a passing waitress and
yelling, "Where's our food!" before we'd even ordered. She
spun the lazy susan around and around, knocking several glasses over. When a big pot of chicken and sweetcorn
soup arrived on the table, she grabbed the closest bowl,
slopped some soup into it, and drank straight from the
rim. She was too drunk to notice that it wasn't a bowl at
all, but an ashtray. *She was drinking soup from an ashtray.*

Our mutual friend, Amy, tried to wrestle it from her

clutches, but she got upset and staggered out of the restaurant, yelling incoherently as she went. Amy and I figured we'd better make sure she got back to her room safely. We hurried after her, but she'd already disappeared into the night. There was no sign of her at the hotel. We spent the next two hours scouring the streets, growing increasingly worried, before finally returning to her room to find her passed out on the bed.

The whole episode freaked me out a bit, so I didn't drink as much as I usually would for the rest of that holiday.

Was I as bad as those two women? They were both single and seemed deeply unhappy. Sure, right now, friends still told me I was a joy; the sparkle and life of the party. But would they want me at their events if I had more episodes like last night? I'd sworn black and blue that Chloé's party was the last time I'd get so out-of-control drunk, and yet, here I was again. Right back to miserable square one.

This pattern was a trap, and for the first time, I could see right through it. This was no way to live; constantly in fear of messing everything up. Why on earth was I self-sabotaging, anyway? I was *this* close to living my dream life, with a new career I was so passionate about and the love-of-my-life by my side. Was I really choosing wine over wellness? Vodka over vitality? Tequila over tranquility?

I suddenly felt incredibly weary, like I'd spent my entire life running. Location changes, career changes, relationship changes. I'd tried it all, and still, that peace and contentment I so desperately craved remained frustratingly out of reach.

A general sensation of dread slowly spread itself across my chest as I had a sickening epiphany. That if I didn't stop drinking, I'd spend the rest of my *life* running.

I couldn't decide which fate was worse; a life spent trying to escape myself, or a sober life. The thought was so unbearable, I started to cry. The grief was all-encompassing and unrelenting. I sobbed heartbreaking tears of sadness for getting myself stuck in this mess. I was supposed to be a health coach. Why couldn't I control this thing?

I didn't want something so stupid to hold me back. I didn't want to feel upset if I couldn't have a drink on Friday nights. I hated that I couldn't even *imagine* a joyful existence without alcohol. I was sick of the anxiety, the shame, and the horrific hangovers slowing me down and keeping me from rocking my passions.

I wanted *freedom,* dammit!

With tears streaming down my face and hands shaking, I flipped open my day planner to the next page and wrote: *If you don't change anything, you don't grow.*

I was afraid of what would happen if I stopped drinking. But I was more afraid of what would happen if I *didn't*.

# FIVE

The next morning, after taking an extraordinary amount of time to get dressed, I finally sat my butt down at my desk and opened my day planner. I knew exactly what I'd written there, but I didn't have the foggiest clue where to begin.

With a deep sigh, I decided on procrastination. I switched on my laptop and scrolled through my Facebook feed. For the first time, I noticed how many photos were of people drinking, or making jokes about needing alcohol to cope with life.

*See?* I reassured myself. *What's the big deal? Everyone binge drinks. It's just a bit of fun.*

Until, of course, it isn't.

Really this whole nonsense should've ended in my twenties. In an ideal world, I would have woken up on my thirtieth birthday and thought, *Wow, that was a blast but I'm so glad I'm mature and sophisticated now. I'm excited to see what comes next, and am so relieved that I can just enjoy a single glass of icy cold Sauvignon Blanc at a dinner party and leave it at that.*

But, no. This had carried on way too far into my thirties, and was becoming increasingly embarrassing. Next year, I'd be staring down the barrel of my fortieth birthday, and then what?

Suddenly, in a very happy flash of synchronicity, I scrolled past a link to an article about the increasing number of 'dry' cafés opening in England. *Wait, what?* I quickly scrolled back and clicked on the link, which opened to show happy people enjoying their lunch sans-alcohol. In the sidebar of the article, I noticed a link to a website called *Soberistas. Cute name*, I thought as I clicked on the link.

All this time, I thought I was alone in this struggle, floundering somewhere along the blurry line between social drinker and alcoholic. But here was a forum created for other women who were struggling with similar issues. What's more, as I continued to click around the site, I saw references to sobriety blogs. I'd written my own wellness blog for the past three years, and yet it had never occurred to me that blogs might exist about sobriety. I'm not sure why that was. Did I really think I was the only woman in the world struggling to put down the glass?

I clicked through to some of the blogs mentioned. As I read through their stories, a shock of recognition ran through me. *The always wanting more, the obsession, the broken 'off' switch.* Other people made drinking rules they couldn't keep, too? Other people felt that all-consuming compulsion to drink more? Other people felt deep levels of shame when their drinking went too far?

Spellbound, I read for hours. Some parts were like a foreign language, but others ripped through my heart like a hurricane, leaving me breathless and dizzy.

As far as I could make out, these women had discovered that it wasn't the third or fourth drink that was the issue for them; it was the very first one. They'd committed to not drinking that first drink, and were chronicling their journey.

Like a suspicious sleuth, I searched the dates of their blog posts and calculated the sums in my head. Some of these bloggers had been sober for many months, some for years. Most reported that they still had tough moments, but overall, their lives were vastly improved by not taking that first drink. Women just like me. Women who previously couldn't imagine a joyful existence without champagne celebrations, cocktails with the girls, and a cheeky Sauvignon Blanc (or seven) with dinner. And they were okay. Heck, more than okay. Here they were, proclaiming that their lives were actually *better* without all that?

My inner critic screamed and pounded against my skull, *Bullshit! They're lying! There's no way!*

My finger itched to close the browser window, but

something stopped me. I mean, why would they lie? And even more mind-blowing; *what if it was true?*

A bubble of hope rose up within me, and my inner critic frantically tried to stick a needle through it. *Can't you just moderate? This is crazy! You don't have to go to such extremes! Everyone drinks! You'll never be invited anywhere. You'll be dull and boring and sit at home, crying into your cornflakes, while everyone else carries on with their romantic, glamorous, wonderful lives.*

For some bizarre reason, one of my favourite scenes from the movie, *The Social Network*, played in my head. It was the part where Mark Zuckerberg spits across the litigation table, "If you guys were the inventors of Facebook, you'd have invented Facebook."

*And if you'd been able to moderate, you would have moderated by now, lady!* All those years spent trying and failing and suffering. All the hangovers, the waking up at 3am, staring at the ceiling, wondering why the hell I kept doing this to myself. My crushed self-esteem, the arguments with my love. Was it all worth it? *Really?*

The previous year, I'd created an ebook for my clients called *The Sparkle Experiment*. This ten-day guide was all about trying healthy new habits and recording how they made you feel. The habits that felt delicious got to stay, and the ones that didn't were chalked up to experience.

What if I thought of *this* as an experiment? You know, just take sobriety for a test drive. If I didn't feel better— if my life wasn't one thousand percent better—I could always drink again. Alcohol wasn't going anywhere anytime soon. I could just try this experiment for a few months and report back to myself. A little health kick of sorts. It'd be good experience for my coaching career anyway, right? I didn't have to become overwhelmed with the magnitude of *forever*. I could just focus on choosing not to drink, right now. Just to see what happens. Because I knew what a drinking life was like. What I didn't know was a sober life.

But how to conduct this experiment? Surely I wasn't 'bad enough' to go to AA. They'd laugh at me; tell me I was being overdramatic. It wasn't like I'd been arrested, lost my job, or crashed my car. I was a woman with a binge drinking issue, that much was clear. But I didn't drink every day, and could sometimes go for ten days or so before I truly missed it. Everyone knew that *real* alcoholics drank all day, every day, right?

So what were the alternatives? Would reading sobriety blogs be enough to get me through it? I thought back to my health coaching studies. We'd covered so many holistic tools to support health and happiness, and I recommended these tools to my clients every day. Yet I still wasn't using many of them myself. Would they be enough to get me through it?

I thought about a 'one hundred day challenge' I'd seen on one of the sobriety blogs. The pledge encouraged making a commitment to reach one hundred days of sobriety, no matter what. Even if it was difficult, or felt shitty, or involved skipping events, or going to bed at 7pm. *No drinking, no matter what.*

This challenge instantly appealed to me. Quite honestly, the thought of never drinking again was terrifying. Even thinking about it caused my chest to constrict and the waterworks to start again.

Months earlier, a friend had invited Dom and I to her 'Christmas in July' dinner party. Still hungover and reeling from another event days prior, I chose not to drink, and the entire night was torturous. Watching other people drink wine and get silly, while I remained seriously sober, was seriously not fun. Not one little bit. Nope, I wasn't ready to even *consider* not drinking again.

*One hundred days.* Three months. Now, that seemed manageable. Long enough to have a proper break and then reassess the situation, but short enough to seem achievable. And a whole lot less scary than *forever*.

I was reading this pledge for about the hundredth time when Dom walked into the study and sat down. "You ok?" he asked. As always, he could sense when I was upset about something.

"Well, I've been reading all these things," I said, swivelling my chair to face him. "I... I think maybe I need to stop drinking for a while. Like, a long while. Like, maybe three months or something."

"Okay..." he said, waiting for me to elaborate, his face hopeful.

"But... that means not drinking on my birthday, and that makes me feel... I just..." Icy fear gripped my chest and I burst into tears. Where was it coming from, all this emotion? I felt more lost than I could ever remember. I was standing on the edge of reason and hope, and I was failing. Failing and flailing.

"Shhh, I'll help you, sweetie. I'm here for you. It's okay. Everything's going to be okay," Dom whispered, pulling me into his arms. As he held me tight, I wished with all my heart that I believed him.

~

Of course, I couldn't let it go without having one final hurrah. One final supper before I walked into what I imagined was a death sentence. The death of life as I knew it.

I'd planned to visit my parents that Friday night, while Dom went out to dinner with his volleyball team. My parents lived an hour away, and there was always wine, so there was never any question that I would stay the night.

As I packed my overnight bag, I felt the usual rush of excitement about seeing them, but there was an underlying feeling of trepidation. Something had shifted in me, and although I hadn't shared any concrete dates or plans with Dom, I knew that this would be my last night of drinking in a long while.

On the drive there, I contemplated starting my sobriety experiment that very minute and declaring it my *Day One*, but the thought depressed me too much. I needed one final session. I wanted one final chance to say goodbye.

My parents were excited to see me, and greeted me with big, warm hugs hello.

"I made your recipe!" Mum said, smiling, as the aroma

of cooked mushrooms enveloped me.

"Oh, it smells amazing," I smiled back.

*Pop!*

"And we've got champagne!" said my Step-Dad, filling our glasses and handing them to us. I guzzled mine greedily, giving myself permission to down as many as I wanted. *If we're gonna' do this, then by Jove, let's do it, good and proper.*

In a New York minute, I was waving my empty champagne flute at my Step-Dad, requesting a refill. As I did, an unwelcome memory barged it's way into my mind, about an ex-boyfriend's Mum. She'd made up a little song that she sang whenever her wine glass was empty, and her husband would dutifully spring up out of his chair to refill it. She sang that song a *lot*. When we visited her, I loved that someone drank as fast, and with as much passion, as I did. Later in the night, she'd become silly and rowdy, and it always embarrassed my ex-boyfriend. He hated it whenever she told us stories of being banned from her local pub for mouthing off at someone, or getting into some other drama. I thought it was hilarious. I loved whenever anyone else got drunk and did stupid things. It took the spotlight off me.

My Step-Dad handed back my glass and I took another big gulp. To my disappointment, it just didn't seem to contain the usual buzz. Try as I might to lift my sagging spirits with glass after glass, the whole process felt tainted with sadness.

I wasn't sure if my parents could tell that something was

off. I charged ahead regardless. Before long, I'd stopped making sense to any of us.

~

The next morning, I woke with a heavy heart and the hangover I deserved. But there was something else there, too. Relief, mixed with something that felt a lot like hope. The line in the sand had been drawn. I was so ready to get out of this ridiculous holding pattern and start feeling better.

Over breakfast, I decided to confide in Mum. I wasn't sure how to bring up the topic, so I just blurted it out. "I hope I didn't keep you up too late last night." I remembered begging her to stay up with me and 'talk more!', but not much after that. She smiled, so I kept going, before I lost my nerve. "I… Um… I'm actually taking a break from drinking for a while." I desperately scanned her face for a reaction. "It's just… all these hangovers, they're killing me. And alcohol is so expensive. And I want to be a good example, for my clients and stuff…"

"Okay," Mum nodded, raising her eyebrows in surprise.

Just then, my Step-Dad walked in from outside where he'd been tinkering with his car. "So when will we see you again?" he asked.

"She's not drinking for a while," Mum told him.

"Aren't you?" he asked, his eyebrows jumping even higher.

"No, I'm… It's a long break. So I can get more stuff

done and not make myself sick all the time…" I fumbled.

"She wants to be a better example for her coaching clients," Mum chimed in to help.

"Oh, okay," my Step-Dad nodded slowly, thinking it over. "Well, you can still see us, can't you?"

"Of course!" I said, even managing a small smile, relieved that I'd survived my first 'non drinking' conversation without having a heart attack.

Later, as I drove away, I remembered the quiet talks Mum had attempted with me at the beginning of each of the three serious relationships I'd had in my life. "Just be careful," she warned, each time she witnessed me acting the drunken fool in front of my love. "You don't want to lose him."

Yep, this decision had been a long time coming and was happening not a day too soon. As I gripped the steering wheel and headed for the freeway, I didn't bother trying not to cry. I was scared, and it wanted to come out, so I let it. For all my mistakes, for all the times I should have stopped drinking but didn't, I sobbed my heart out.

~

"Today's *Day One*," I announced to Dom as I walked through the front door.

"Oh, that's awesome!" he smiled, jumping up from the couch and kissing me. He paused. "Wait. So that means, tomorrow…"

"I won't be drinking," I declared, with much more conviction than I felt. Right smack-bang in the middle of 'Day Two', I had Brooke's hens party to attend. Thankfully it was an afternoon high tea event and not the traditional drunken affair. I figured I could eat enough cake to get me through it without champagne. "I'll drive, and I'll take cake, and I'll be really proud of myself when I get back," I said, as much for Dom as for my own ears.

"And I'll be proud of you," Dom said.

I nodded my hungover head. It hurt like hell. I remembered a comment a woman had made on one of the sobriety blogs. At a hen's party, her friend had remarked, "Oh, it's so good that you can come out with us, even though you're not drinking!" To which, the woman replied, "*Jeez*, I'm sober, not dying!" I had a good chuckle when I read it, but part of me was worried that I'd be greeted with the same kind of reaction. A sober, non-pregnant woman, at a hens party? It was unheard of!

I headed to the kitchen and pulled ingredients from the cupboard, determined to make a delicious chocolate slice to take with me. Following a vegan lifestyle hadn't really been a problem for me in social situations before. I'd always just focused on the alcohol and found something to eat when I got home. Now that alcohol would be out of the picture, I'd need to be vigilant about taking food with me. Even if I wasn't hungry, I knew I'd crave the distraction.

As I mixed and stirred, I tried to tell the butterflies in my stomach that this wholesome lifestyle was going to be fun. No hangovers, no walks of shame, no texting sheepish apologies to friends.

The butterflies weren't buying it.

~

I woke up the next morning feeling much better. Day One was over, thank God, and the majority of my hangover had disappeared with it. I was still nervous about this sobriety challenge, but with a clear head I felt more optimistic, and even more determined to view it as a big adventure.

I took my time getting ready, knowing that if I was happy with how I looked, I'd feel more confident. I to'd and fro'd between wearing something plain and simple, to fade into the background, or wearing something bold and fun to cheer me up. Finally, I decided on the latter. In a bright fuchsia dress, there was no chance of me being a wallflower, but it felt more festive and appropriate. At the very least, it might provide a talking point to distract from the lack of alcohol in my glass.

On the drive over, I mentally high-fived myself. *Check out this mature, sophisticated woman, driving to her friend's hens party! If someone drinks too much and gets embarrassingly silly today, for once it won't be me!*

Had I been drinking, I would have spent the entire cab ride giving myself a lecture that it was okay to be enthusiastic about the drinks, as long as I didn't go overboard. Now I was giving myself a pep talk in the other direction; that it was okay to be sober. *My first sober hens party.* To distract myself from freaking out, I turned up the radio and attempted to sing along to the girly tunes.

I found a handy parking spot right outside the brides-maid's house. As my high heels clicked up the path to the front door, the butterflies stretched their wings again. *Pesky little critters.* I knocked on the front door and attempted to breathe normally.

"Hiiii! Come on in!" sang a woman I didn't recognise, swinging the door wide open. "We're out the back."

I followed her to the back garden. It was gorgeous. The patio was decorated with balloons in pastel colours and delicate hanging ornaments. Multiple cake stands lined the white tablecloths. I found an empty stand towards the back, and set down the chocolate slice I'd made.

"Hi chick!" Melissa said, coming up to hug me hello. "We're over here." She motioned to four of our friends standing amongst the twenty or so well-dressed ladies on the patio.

"Champagne?" Louise asked after we'd all hugged our greetings.

"Um… I might just have a juice," I said, far more awkwardly than I'd hoped. "I'll get it." I spun on my heels and made a beeline for the buffet tables. I figured pouring my own drink had the double benefit of giving me a chance to pull myself together, and ensuring that no-one accidentally handed me a champagne and orange juice combo.

"Did you drive?" Melissa asked as I rejoined the group, her eyes scanning my glass. I'd poured the juice into a champagne flute, but it was so completely out of character for me not to be drinking, it was only natural that she asked.

"Yep, I did," I nodded. I tried to be cool about it, but my cheeks betrayed me. Oh well, I might as well get this conversation over with early. "I… I'm not drinking for a while."

"What… Forever?" she asked, not seeming all that surprised.

"Uh… Well, we'll see…" I stammered.

"Or just for a month or something?" Alice prompted.

I felt my blush deepen as all eyes turned to me. "Well, I was thinking more like three months or so…"

"Oh, okay," Melissa and Alice nodded in unison, causing me to wonder if they'd all been talking about me, swapping stories about what a horrible drunk I was, and wondering when I'd finally come to my senses.

Ashleigh swiftly changed the subject, making me feel even more paranoid. Had they suspected this was coming after my performance at the last couple of events? Or was not drinking for three months truly no big deal to them? I certainly couldn't remember anyone ever stopping for months at a time. Even fundraising initiatives like *Dry July* always seemed to cause shockwaves on the social scene. Every year, I witnessed truckloads of my Facebook friends white-knuckling it through the month, begging other friends to buy them 'night out' passes so they didn't have to face a whole month without booze.

I was relieved that the conversation had moved on, but ashamed that it had come to this; that complete sobriety felt like the only answer. And yet, there was still a beautiful mixture of relief and hope in there, too. The endless attempts to moderate my drinking were freaking *exhausting,* and I was surprised to find I was actually looking forward to taking an extended break.

I could only hope, with enough time, everyone would forget my messiest shenanigans and come to see me in a new light. And most of all, that I'd see *myself* in that new light. It was well overdue.

# SIX

The next day, I woke up feeling liberated. Like I'd narrow-
ly escaped wrongful imprisonment. Waking up without a
hangover—or a heart full of regret—felt utterly delicious,
and the thought of not having to deal with another one for
three whole months was sublime. I hummed and danced
my way through the morning, feeling incredibly pleased
with myself. Any other hens party would have seen me re-
covering on the couch the entire next day. *Not this time,
my friend,* I thought smugly, *not this time.*

The last hens party I went to was Ashleigh's, years earlier. That night ended with me being so incoherently drunk,
Melissa had called Dom to come and collect me from the

bar. It was the right thing to do, of course, but even so, I couldn't help feeling hurt. Like they'd betrayed me by working together. Like alcohol and I were on one side, and they were on the other.

Well, there was going to be none of that nonsense for the next few months. My reputation and I were going to be squeaky clean for a change.

I'd learnt an important lesson over the previous few years, first in adopting a vegan lifestyle, then going gluten-free, then launching a wellness business from scratch. It was that having a great toolbox of support could mean the difference between weeping alone in the corner, and rocking it out and actually *enjoying* the challenge. Before embarking on a lifestyle change of this magnitude, I knew I'd need help, and lots of it.

Before next weekend arrived, I was going to need a serious Action Plan.

Back when I was in my corporate job, we were encouraged to take a 'Defensive Driving' course that involved performing a variety of manoeuvres on a race track. In one of the exercises, we were instructed to speed up and then slam on the brakes and avoid hitting a particular safety cone. Despite our best efforts, we all hit that cone.

We tried the activity again, but this time, rather than focusing on the cone, we were instructed to look for a safe place to steer the car. Same distance, same speed, same brakes; just a different intention and focus.

We were stunned. Every single one of us avoided the cone.

Our instructor explained that if something or someone jumps out in front of you, the worst thing you can do is look straight at it as you're trying to avoid it. You need to focus on where you *want* to go, rather than where you *don't* want to go.

The lesson was powerful and I often found myself telling clients about it. Time and again, I noticed that when we focus on our fears, we often smash into them. And if we're not focusing on where we really want to go, how can we expect to get there?

I thought about the next three months and everything I wanted to do, see, hear, taste, and experience in that time. Above all, I thought about how I wanted to *feel*. I wanted to feel playful, with confidence that was authentically *me*, not poured from a bottle. I wanted deeper connections, less anxiety, more space, more love, more potential. I wanted *transformation*, dammit!

I didn't want to undertake a challenge that would make me miserable, and I was determined to make this experience a positive one. Sensing that overwhelm was not my friend, I decided to start with just two words of intention that inspired me most. I opened my journal to a fresh page, and wrote, *My Sobriety Experiment*.

My biggest fear around sobriety was that I'd never have fun again, so I decided to start with the big one. On the next line, I wrote, *Playful*. I thought about what playful meant to me. *Creativity, fun, spontaneity, mischief, joy.*

I tapped my pen against the page, thinking about what I could do to feel that way without booze. I brainstormed on the page:

*Choose love over fear. Trust. Believe. Tell jokes. Send funny messages to friends. Tickle Dom. Make fun demo videos. Create fun, easy recipes. Schedule time off-line. Watch funny movies. View each day as an adventure. Try new things. Take beautiful photos. Invite friends to lunch. Paint my toe nails. Create. Share. Skip. Giggle. Dance.*

I took a deep breath as I reviewed my list. *See?* I told my inner critic. *That doesn't sound so bad.*

I turned the page and chose my next word, *Radiant.* I thought about what that word meant to me. *Sparkly, healthy, glowing, connected, blissful.* Obviously, just skipping the alcohol would guarantee that I felt infinitely more radiant, but what else could I do? I jotted down everything that came to mind:

*Stretch before bed. Go to bed earlier. Stretch at sunrise. Juice. Run. Go to yoga class. Offer help. Eat plenty of fresh, whole foods. Feel sunshine on my skin. Splash around at the beach. Picnic in the park. Keep a gratitude journal. Meditate. Write. Create. Eat dinner by candlelight. Choose quality over quantity. Phone friends and family. Listen. Practice random acts of kindness.*

I reviewed my lists, and started to feel tingles of excitement about this little adventure. Inspired, I switched on my laptop and created a secret Mood Board on Pinterest. I wanted something pretty I could look at on my phone whenever I felt shaky; images to remind me how I wanted to *feel*, and why I was doing this. Why I wanted to change; what life might be like without this unhealthy habit; the kind of person I could become if I were free of its clutches.

Like a woman possessed, I spent hours clicking around the internet. Nutritious food, women doing yoga, women running on the beach, women splashing around in the ocean, *click click click*.

Job done, and feeling marginally better about the whole endeavour, I decided to go one step further. I had a feeling this challenge would be one of the biggest of my life and I'd need all the safety nets I could possibly create.

For my birthday the previous year, Dom bought me the large vision board I'd been swooning over for months. It was gorgeous, with a huge expanse of white space to pin pictures, and a beautiful wooden frame, painted white. He'd kept it a surprise, filling the board with photos from our travels and other meaningful souvenirs. He snuck it into our study before coming in to meet me and a huge group of friends at a bar in the city. Naturally, because it was my birthday, I got rather silly indeed, downing cocktail after cocktail like it was the eve of Prohibition.

Dom had planned to surprise me with his thoughtful gift when we got home that night, but my actions robbed him, and myself, of the chance. I was a drunken mess and didn't even remember the cab ride home. The next morning, when he took me into our study and showed it to me, I felt wretched with guilt and stupidity.

Now, I took a deep breath and lifted the board off the

wall. It was time for an update; to the board, and to my *life*. I fixed a vision in my mind of the sexy, sober woman I wanted to be. Then, just as I'd done with my Pinterest board, I filled the board with images aligned with that vision, this time cut from magazines.

Three hours later, I was finally done.

On a roll now, and proud of myself for being so thorough in my preparations, I opened my laptop and signed up to an Australian website called *Hello Sunday Morning*. Similar to *Soberistas,* this was another forum where people undergoing similar challenges in redefining their relationship with alcohol could share their stories and encourage each other. I certainly wasn't brave enough to share my own experiences just yet, but even the act of joining the site and publicly stating my 'three month' intentions—albeit using an alias—felt like a monumental leap.

Next, I clicked over to my favourite online bookstore and ordered a copy of Jason Vale's book, '*Kick the Drink… Easily!*'. I still wasn't convinced that I'd do it *easily*, but many sober bloggers reported that the book made a lot of valid points and could help the reader to see things differently, and therefore, succeed in breaking the habits of a lifetime. It was worth a try.

Lastly, I downloaded a 'day tracker' app onto my phone and decided that one hundred days was my goal. The fact that this idea terrified me, only made me all the more determined to actually follow through this time.

"What are you up to, sweetie? Is everything okay?" Dom asked, appearing in the doorway when I still hadn't emerged from the study at dinner time.

"It's more than okay," I smiled at him. I showed him my action plan, inspirations, and vision boards.

"Very cool," he laughed, looking it all over. He stared at the updated vision board on the wall. I wondered if he was thinking about the previous year when I'd ruined my birthday surprise. He pulled me closer to him. "I'm going to do the challenge with you."

"What?" I stared at him. "Really? But… Are you sure? You don't have to." The idea that anyone would voluntarily give up alcohol floored me.

"Of course I'm sure," he smiled, his mind already made up. "Three months. You and me."

Tears filled my eyes as gratitude swirled through me. *This is why I'm doing it*, I reminded myself as I looked up at him. *This is love.*

With Dom by my side, I felt stronger and more determined, but deep down I knew this challenge was mine alone. Even if he changed his mind, I needed to keep going. Three months. *No matter what.*

As I climbed into bed that night, I couldn't help but smile. With my sober tool belt, I felt much more confident and optimistic.

Now it was time for the true test; how to make it as a sober woman in the big, wide world.

~

An invitation to Mark and Brooke's wedding presented me with my first chance to practice. It was Saturday night, and just Day 8 of my little experiment.

I spent longer than usual getting ready, once again convinced that looking good would give me the confidence boost I needed to actually get my butt out the door. Those pesky butterflies were at it again.

"Shall we order a cab?" I called out to Dom as I put the hairdryer away.

"No," he laughed, appearing in the bathroom doorway. "We'll drive."

"Oh yeah," I said with a nervous laugh.

This was a wedding cocktail party. What would people think about me not drinking? How many questions would I have to deal with? More importantly, how long would we have to stay?

In the car on the drive over, I practiced taking slow, steady breaths.

"You'll be fine, sweetie," Dom reassured me, reaching over to squeeze my hand.

I thought about the raw chocolate treat I'd made earlier that day, and strategically placed in the freezer as a reward for myself when I got home. I thought about how great I'd feel the next morning. Then the nerves hit. *God, I hope I make it through this thing alive.*

We arrived to find the place already jumping. It was the hottest new bar in town, freshly renovated with funky industrial lighting. Long, polished wooden tables reflected the lights around the room, giving the whole bar a warm glow. Although the mood was lively, the bar wasn't as crowded as I'd expected, and for that I thanked my lucky stars. Still, I felt out of place. When was the last time I'd been sober at a cocktail party or wedding?

We spotted a group of our friends standing around one of the tables and hugged them hello.

"Go get some drinks!" Meghan said, gesturing towards the bar. "There's a tab."

Dom held my hand as he led the way. "Let's get mocktails," he said, smiling and reaching for a menu. He was trying to make the event as easy and fun as he could for me, and I loved him for it. I let him choose our drinks, while my eyes scanned the bottles lining the wall behind the bartender. Small, strategically placed lights caused the bottles to sparkle.

*Why the hell can't I just have a few drinks and have a good time? It's not fair!* I felt like wailing, but forced myself to take another shaky breath. *Remember your Action Plan.*

The drinks took an age. When the bartender finally handed me a tall tiki mug, I took a long sip. It was delicious; nice and sour, just the way I like them. I smiled at Dom, delighted with his choice.

*See?* I told myself, as we headed back to our friends. *It's only a hundred days. You'll live.*

The bar grew louder as the clock ticked onwards and more people poured in. Women sloshed wine out of their glasses as they hugged their friends hello, and I tried not to feel sick with envy. *Focus on the good stuff,* I reminded myself. I took another deep breath and turned towards Louise. "How was your week, hon?" I asked.

"Good," she smiled. "What's that?" She pointed at my tiki mug.

"It's a mocktail," I told her, attempting a smile that came out more like a grimace.

"Wow," she said. "At a wedding. You're so strong."

"Yeah," I mumbled and stared at my shoes, feeling exactly the opposite. When she reached out and touched my arm, it was almost my undoing. Like when you're upset about something, but manage to hold it together until someone asks tenderly, "Are you okay?" And then you melt into a puddle on the floor.

"Hey Bex," Ashleigh interrupted, coming up beside me. I turned to her, grateful for the distraction. "Can you taste this?" She shoved her drink in front of my nose. "Does it have alcohol in it? Liam ordered me a mocktail but it smells like it has alcohol." Ashleigh was four months pregnant, so I understood why she was worried, but I didn't know what to do. Louise had already turned to talk to someone else. I stared at the glass, just inches from my face. "I… Umm…" I stammered, trying to smother my impending panic attack.

I'd told the girls about this sobriety challenge at Brooke's hens party the weekend before, but I realised now, they couldn't possibly understand what it entailed. In their minds, it was just a sip, for God's sake. *What's the big deal?*

But I knew it *was* a big deal. I knew if I took one sip, I'd want more. I'd see it as a free pass; an excuse to go nuts that night. I'd be cheating on the whole challenge and have to start all over again. Was it worth it?

Sensing my rising panic, Dom swooped in and grabbed the glass.

"Nope!" he said cheerfully after taking a sip. "All good." He handed the glass back to Ashleigh. Relief and gratitude rushed through me, making me giddy. Once again, to my utter frustration, I felt like crying. Was it going to be this hard *all the freaking time?*

I thought back to a few months earlier when I'd met Ashleigh for lunch after one of my particularly drunken episodes. I was the first to arrive at the café and saved us a table. When she joined me, I greeted her with a sheepish grin. "I'm sorry about last night," I said, before she even had a chance to sit down.

"What? Oh, you were fine, hon," she said, waving away my concern. "We've all been there."

"Yeah," I nodded. "I seem to go there the most, though." A deep shame spread through my veins, making me feel hot and cold at the same time. I didn't know whether to attempt to laugh it off, or burst into tears. Hiding under the table suddenly seemed like a brilliant idea.

"Well, look," she said, her eyes scanning my face. "Maybe you could slow down a bit. I always have a water between my drinks. Maybe you could try that too? Plus, I drink slowly. Why don't you try pacing yourself with me?" I nodded, but in my heart I knew that I'd been trying those methods for years. Some nights they worked. Most nights they didn't.

So now I was trying sobriety and hoping that it would

'work'. That I'd finally find some sense of peace. Because what other option was there? Moderation, madness, or sobriety. Pick one and hope to hell you find what you're looking for.

But seriously, *three months of this?* I didn't think I could take it. I did my best to smile and pretend I was having a good time, but inside, I was miserable. My feet hurt, the bar was so loud, and I just wanted to go home.

By 11pm, Dom could see I was struggling to hold it together. "Let's go," he whispered in my ear. I'd never heard two words more magical in all my life.

As we walked back to the car, I didn't care about my action plan, or the raw chocolate waiting for me in the freezer, or how great I'd feel the next day. I just couldn't wait to crawl into bed and rethink this whole thing.

# SEVEN

The next morning, I woke up feeling deflated and irritable. "I'm never going out again," I announced to Dom.

"It was just the first one," he chuckled. "It'll get easier."

As I shuffled about the apartment, getting dressed and making breakfast, I turned the whole thing over in my mind. Clearly, I was going to have to double-down on my tools if I wanted to make it through this whole sobriety experiment with my sanity intact.

The problem with drinking for so long is that I'd forgotten what I used to enjoy doing, before wine came along. For decades, my definition of fun was any activity that involved alcohol. Never mind that it all came with a mountain of negative consequences. In my mind, drinking was fun. Period.

I plopped myself down at my desk to think about it. What made me happy? What were some small things could I do to cheer myself up? I opened my journal to a fresh page. At the top, I wrote, *My Self-Love & Kindness Menu.*

I started brainstorming, jotting down everything I could think of:

*Curling up in bed with a good book. Lighting a scented candle. Taking a long bubble bath. Cooking a fancy meal. Putting fresh sheets on the bed.*

*Hmm,* I thought. *Not enough. What else?*

I continued scribbling:

*Going to new bookstores, theatres, plays, and foreign films. Dancing around the apartment to my favourite songs. Girly catch-ups over brunch. Blissfully sleeping in.*

I paused to re-read my list. Feeling marginally better, I vowed to do at least one of these things for myself each week. They'd give me something to look forward to, in addition to the little gifts I'd give myself each day. I decided to channel all the money I usually spent on wine and taxi fares into things like fresh flowers, new books, and raw chocolate. Not to mention, drinking a ton of sparkling mineral water in fancy crystal goblets, and hugging Dom a lot. Basically, anything I could think of to make this whole sobriety challenge more like an adventure, and less like an act of torture.

~

Proving that how I did one thing was how I did everything, I promptly became addicted to reading every sobriety blog and article I could find. I clicked deep into the archives, reading each blogger's account of their first three months. Inhaling every tiny detail like I'd once inhaled wine.

"How's it going, sweetie?" Dom said, finding me in the study with my face pressed up against the computer screen.

"Some of it's still jibberish to me," I told him. "But it's all fascinating. They talk about things called 'pink clouds' and a 'wolf', but I haven't been able to figure out what they're referring to yet."

"Okay," he smiled, leaving me to it. "I'll make us some tea."

All this research provided a welcome distraction, and I loved every minute of it. I clicked around for another hour or so, before finding more about the 'wolf' character they were all so familiar with. It seemed to be inspired by the *Bad Wolf* parable; that we all have a 'good wolf' and a 'bad wolf' battling for power within us. Light and dark. Love and fear. The wolf who wins is the one we 'feed' by listening to it, and acting on it.

I leaned back in my chair as I had a huge *'a-ha'* moment. It was the same principle as all the spiritual books I'd ever read, and everything I taught my clients about our constant choice between love and fear. It all made sense. The ego ran on fear. It was afraid of our old identity dying, and would do or say anything to keep us 'safe' in our current state, even if it was excruciating. *Better the devil you know.*

Some bloggers labelled the 'bad wolf', 'Wolfie', while others called it the 'Wine Witch' or 'addict voice'. I loved the idea of giving that voice a name. To know the enemy, and to have a character to brace myself against. I knew I'd hate myself less, and look after myself more, knowing that all those empty promises and manipulative thoughts weren't coming from my heart or spirit, but from my addict voice. All those sick whispers, *You can just have one, you weren't that bad, you're making life hard for yourself, you don't really have a problem anyway.* They were lies; the taunts of a desperate beast. One book explained that 'telling on' the voice was a great way to challenge its authority over our brains, and rob it of its power.

Dom walked in with another pot of tea, and I told him everything I'd discovered.

"Okay," he nodded, thinking it over. "You tell me what the beast says, and I'll help you stay focused on the truth."

"Really?" When we'd launched into this entrepreneurial lifestyle, I was blessed to find that Dom was an incredible coach. I trusted him completely and knew I could be honest with him, but this felt like a scary new level of vulnerability. He didn't know the kind of cruel nonsense that voice said to me.

"Really," he confirmed with a smile. "We're in this together."

I exhaled nervously. I was willing to give it a try. "Well, right *now*, the beast is telling me I'm craving a drink."

"But that's not the truth," he reminded me. "What are you *really* craving?" It was a question he'd heard me ask my clients many times, encouraging them to dig deeper into what was really going on.

It was a conversation we'd repeat many times over the following months. On good days, having Dom in my corner made me feel like I could move mountains, and I didn't think it was possible for one human to love another more. On bad days, it infuriated me. *I'm craving a god-damned drink,* I wanted to scream, stamping my foot while I was at it. Instead, I threw myself on our bed and sobbed. Bucket loads of tears. Wallowing in my pity party until I made myself sick with misery.

At night, I tuned in to sobriety podcasts. I also read countless addiction memoirs, but was disappointed that most of them ended when the author stopped drinking. As though that was the end of the story of their lives.

Which, of course, was exactly what I was afraid of.

~

On Day 15, I met Holly for brunch at Solomon's—the same café from the day of the Earth Angel event. I arrived a few minutes early and chose one of the cute outdoor tables in the sunshine. As I sat down to wait, it occurred to me just how insanely tired I was. It had been a big week. Obviously, there was my emotional turmoil after finding the wedding cocktail party so difficult to navigate. We'd also just relaunched *The Sparkle Project*, so my week had been filled with client sessions. But this felt like a new level of exhaustion. If I didn't know any better, I'd say it was my body detoxing.

I sat up straight in my chair. *It couldn't be a physical detox, could it? I'd only been drinking a few nights per week, not every day.*

I thought about how my body had taken a good thirty days to detox from dairy, and then again from gluten, and realised how naïve I'd been. I should have seen this coming.

A year or so earlier, I'd tried a raw food cleanse and remembered Louise saying, "*Ooh*, I read that something like eighty percent of all people who eat a raw food diet stop drinking." She paused, letting that statistic sink in. "So be *careful!*"

"Oh, that'll never happen, don't worry!" I assured her and we fell about, giggling like teenagers.

I wished I had the motivation to try that raw diet again to see if it helped, but it was all I could do to keep myself from spending half the day elbow deep in the cookie jar. I knew that green juice always made me feel better, and I'd been drinking as much juice as I could. But more often that not, a sugary treat won out instead. I knew this wasn't helping my cause one little bit, but I figured it was the lesser of two evils. *Better sugar than alcohol for now*, I reasoned. I vowed to order a green juice as soon as Holly arrived.

Just then, I spotted her hurrying along the footpath towards me. I smiled and waved, excited to see her.

"Hi babe!" she called, waving back. We hugged hello, and I handed her a menu as she settled into the seat opposite me.

Although we hadn't been friends for long, I knew she had a warm, caring nature. In that moment, I decided to confide in her. "Well," I announced awkwardly. "I haven't had a drink in two weeks."

"Cool," she smiled in a casual way, like it was truly no big deal. As if I'd simply told her that I switched my breakfasts from chia puddings to smoothie bowls.

I paused, wondering whether to just change the subject. She looked at me.

"Oh," she said, as the penny dropped. "Is that quite challenging for you, babe?"

"Yeah," I blushed. "Well… Um… Remember after the Earth Angel event? When you said all that alcohol talk was boring?"

"Uh huh," she nodded, not taking her eyes off me.

"Well, it really resonated with me. Because… I drink too much."

"Do you?" she asked, her eyes widening in surprise. I realised just how well I'd compartmentalised my life. My drinking friends couldn't imagine me sober, and my wellness friends couldn't imagine me drunk.

"Yeah," I admitted.

"So how's it going?"

"Well," I paused to gather my thoughts. I wanted to start on a positive note. "Some days I feel amazing and whizz around, making a ton of healthy snacks, and going for long walks. I sleep better, and waking up without a hangover is *so freaking good*. It never gets old." I smiled. "And I've fallen in love with herbal tea. I've filled our cupboard with all different kinds. Chamomile, peppermint, green, jasmine, lemongrass…" As someone who'd never particularly cared for tea, this new ritual fascinated me.

"But it's been tough, too," I continued. "Some days I feel like a total basket case. I've been tired, and overly emotional. I've even thrown a tantrum or two. Poor Dom."

"I so can't imagine you throwing a tantrum," she said, shaking her head.

"*Ooh*, it's not pretty," I said, scrunching up my face, and we both laughed.

I changed the subject, asking Holly about her recent holiday, and how her work was going. It was heavenly to have a break from thinking about sobriety for a while. But later, when Holly went inside to fetch the dessert menus, I wondered exactly *why* I'd been so emotional without alcohol.

When I was twenty-seven and working in Sydney, a new girl joined our team. She was in her early twenties, petite, and very quiet. One day, as I was trying—and failing—to stifle a giggle at a joke one of my team mates had emailed me, I caught her staring at me.

"You are the most cheerful person I've ever met," she said, with a look I could only describe as awe.

Later that week, she pulled me aside to tell me that she'd been to see her doctor. "I've been feeling so stressed out," she explained. "My husband likes to run the house a certain way, and I like it a different way, and I don't know how to deal with it, and then I get so angry and upset."

"Oh, hon." I took her hands in mine. She was so young,

and as many cultures dictate, she'd only left her parent's house and moved in with her love after their honeymoon. It was all so new.

"The doctor said I need a stress outlet. He said everybody has one, and I need to figure out what mine will be. So I wanted to ask you, because you're always happy, what's *your* stress outlet?"

"Oh," I said, caught completely off guard. "Wine," I laughed, then seeing her earnest face and knowing she wasn't much of a drinker, I added, "Exercise is usually the best way, hon. Why don't you see if a girlfriend wants to play tennis with you? Or take up running, or a fun dance class?"

I thought I was joking about wine being my coping mechanism, but now I wondered how much truth was in it. Could I cope with stress without alcohol? Or, as many of my sobriety books suggested, had my inner growth been stunted at around the same time I'd taken up drinking?

*Was is it possible that I had the emotional maturity of a sixteen year old?*

~

The next morning I woke up feeling raw and exposed. When had I allowed alcohol to become such a crutch? I had to learn to stand on my own two feet. Deciding to face it head-on, I marched into the bathroom and stood before the mirror. *A grown woman should know how to soothe herself without falling into the bottle*, I told my reflection. I took a deep breath and tapped on my chest with the first three fingers of each hand. As I looked into my eyes, I repeated, "I choose sobriety. I choose happiness."

This 'tapping' process was also known as Emotional Freedom Technique, or EFT. It was a healing tool based on ancient Chinese acupressure and modern psychology that I'd learnt about from the many wellness websites I followed. The practice involved 'tapping' on specific energy meridian points around the body while repeating affirmations. It was supposed to be highly effective at busting through limiting beliefs and negative patterns—including addiction.

When I first heard about it, I thought it sounded pretty kooky, but I tried it anyway. As instructed, I repeated phrases like, *"Even though I'm worried about [insert worry here], I know that I'm [insert affirmation here], and I completely love and accept myself."* It felt very odd at first, but I was thrilled to discover how powerful it was in soothing my anxiety.

Now, I wondered why on earth I hadn't continued to use it. It felt like visiting an old friend.

That night, I read more sobriety blogs and books. "The bloggers talk about something called 'sober momentum'," I told Dom when he came to bed. "They say the more days you accumulate in a row, the easier sobriety becomes. And that momentum is very precious, because it's much harder to stop drinking the second time around."

"Good thing you're only doing it once then," he said. I pulled a face. *One could only hope.*

Whenever I started to wonder if I was just being extreme, I read through the comments on those blogs. I liked that they scared me. So many women before me had thought exactly the same thing, only to find that they were, in fact, *that bad*. That they couldn't magically drink in moderation, simply because they'd had a long period of sobriety. They wrote about the heartache of finding themselves back at square one, but with their lives now even more damaged, because their self-esteem had taken a monumental beating.

Deep down, I knew that freedom would never come from trying to moderate. Because it was a slippery slope of bad decisions. If I could justify drinking at a wedding, why not a birthday? And if I could justify drinking on Friday and Saturday, Sunday wouldn't be far behind. Nope, true freedom would only come from never wanting to drink that poison again. I understood this, and most days I could remind myself of it and feel okay, but some days were just a whole lot harder than others.

The sobriety blogs promised I'd feel remarkably better after 60 days. So most nights, I went to bed at 7 or 8pm and hid under the covers, seeking sweet relief from the noise in my head and the pain in my heart. Wishing, with every fibre of my being, for Day 60 to hurry the hell up.

~

On Day 17, Louise and I had plans to visit our friend Cara. We hadn't seen her for weeks, since she'd given birth to her first baby, a darling little girl.

"What did you make?" Louise asked as I climbed into her car, holding a basket.

"Chickpea curry. Not too spicy. You?"

"Ooh, she'll love it. I made a veggie bake thing. It's really yummy," she said, pulling away from the verge. Figuring the first few months of motherhood would be hectic, we'd agreed to bring meals that Cara could reheat for dinner on the nights she felt too exhausted to cook.

When we arrived, Cara swung the door open. She was thrilled to see us—and even more excited when we handed her the meals. "Come in!" she smiled. "Have a seat."

We got comfy on her couch and chatted about baby life, before Cara asked out of the blue, "So Bex, are you not drinking?"

I felt my cheeks flush. "No… Um, I'm not." I glanced at Louise. She stared back at me.

"For how long?" Cara persisted.

"Uh, I think a couple of months at least. Just to have a long break. Until I get my head straight," I fumbled.

"Not forever, though," said Louise. It wasn't a question.

"Well… maybe…" I replied.

Louise stared at me, horrified. My cheeks burned even hotter.

"It's just not good for me, Louise," I explained. "I always get so embarrassingly smashed—so much drunker than everyone else—and I feel sick, awful, and anxious, for *days*. I can't cope with it anymore."

"But, you can just slow down…" she suggested.

I sighed. "Hon, I drank every bottle of wine in your house when I house-sat for you. I had to go to the bottle store the day before you came back, frantically trying to replace them all. I did the same when I house-sat for Bronwyn. It's exhausting, and it's not normal."

"Oh," she said, still looking unconvinced.

"I can completely relate, Bex," Cara said, rocking her baby. "I'm glad I've got this little one to keep me out of trouble now. Before I got pregnant, I did a lot of things I'm not proud of. I attracted a lot of drama, and I know most of it wouldn't have happened if I didn't drink so much."

We were all quiet for a moment, before Louise changed the subject, and I began to breathe normally again. In a strange way, it felt good to get it all out in the open. But all this truth and vulnerability was so *intense*. Sobriety should come with an oxygen tank. No wonder I was so exhausted all the time. It was an emotional freaking rollercoaster.

# EIGHT

The following afternoon, I was sitting on the couch, scrolling through Facebook. I'd always loved joining in on the banter, so it was strange to find that I couldn't cope. Seeing everyone else out drinking with their friends was doing my head in. Every time I saw a photo of a smiling group holding their glasses up in a toast, I lost my shit.

I put my phone away and attempted to shake off the icky feeling. *Old Bex would be there with them*, the beast snarled.

*Yes, and Old Bex would drink too much and make herself sick*, I shot back. I stomped to the bathroom. I tried saying affirmations into the mirror.

The beast piped up again. *Why do you have to make life so hard for yourself? You're going to regret missing out on all these good times.*

*No, I'm not!* I declared, staring at my reflection. *I've been doing that stuff for twenty years. I'm going to make a better life for myself, and I'm going to have even better times.*

*With zero friends,* the beast sneered.

"Aaarrggg!" I groaned out loud, marching back to the kitchen.

"What's *wrong*?" Dom asked, noticing my disgusting mood. "Have you been on Facebook again?"

"Yes," I grumbled. He knew me too well.

"Well, I can't help you if you won't help yourself," he scoffed, and walked away. I crossed my arms and sulked. He was right, of course, but that didn't make it any less infuriating.

"For God's sake!" I huffed, ever the drama queen. But I knew what I had to do. Facebook was obviously a huge trigger for me, and if I was determined to maintain a positive mindset, it had to go. I reached for my phone and deleted the app.

Still feeling awful and anxious, I wondered what I could do to make myself feel better. In a flash of inspiration, I headed for the study. Shuffling through the bookshelf, I finally found it. The handmade journal with the gold cover; the one I'd been saving for something special.

I sat at my desk and flipped to the first page. At the top, I wrote: *My Gratitude Journal.* I paused, thinking it over. What was I grateful for? I scribbled two things that immediately came to mind:

*Morning sunshine in our apartment with my Love. Client told me our session helped her to see things differently.*

I took a deep breath. Despite mood swings that gave me whiplash, I knew I had so much to be thankful for. I vowed that whenever I felt tempted to scroll through Facebook, I'd write in my gratitude journal instead.

Feeling pleased with myself for outsmarting the beast, I went to find Dom. He was working on something at his computer. "I'm feeling better now," I told him. He looked up, waiting for me to elaborate. With a shy smile, I filled him in on the details.

"I'm proud of you," he hugged me. "How about we go to dinner to celebrate? Superstar Thai?" It was a nickname we'd given to our favourite Thai restaurant. The food was amazing, but really, it held a special place in my heart because they stocked my favourite champagne.

"We'll get those fresh coconut juices," he said, reading my mind. An image of a pretty orchid peeking out of a festive glass danced in my head, instantly cheering me up. It'd feel strange, not drinking there. I'd only ever loved going out to dinner for the wine. But this was part of the process, right? Flexing my sober muscles in different situations.

I smiled. "Let's go."

~

On Day 19, I met Sophie for a celebratory birthday lunch. We were born just nine days apart, and throughout our twenty-five year friendship, we'd often had private lunch parties—just the two of us—in addition to celebrations with family and friends. We typically went to a pub or licensed café for a cheeky glass of chardonnay with our lunch, but I told her I wasn't in the mood and wanted to go to a regular café.

"This is so weird, having a birthday lunch without wine. Are you *sure*?" she asked as we walked in.

"Yep," I said stiffly, and attempted a small smile. There was no need for me to be so awkward with Sophie, but I couldn't help it. When I didn't elaborate, She gave me a funny sideways look, like, *You weirdo*. I wanted to wait until we were seated before things got all hot and heavy with explanations.

We placed our orders at the counter and found a small table in the alfresco section out the front. The café was right near the entrance to the shopping mall, and we watched people come and go, pushing trolleys and strollers and tugging children along.

*This isn't so weird*, I told myself. *It's the middle of the day. What do we need alcohol for?*

Truthfully, I missed it, and I was pretty sure Sophie missed it too. "I actually think I'm going to stop drinking for a while, hon," I said as soon as we sat down, my heart pounding against my rib cage. No point prolonging the agony. May as well get it out there before the food arrived.

"Like, a health kick or something?" she asked. "For how long?"

"Well, I'm not sure yet. It's been nineteen days so far." I paused for effect. Just as I'd predicted, she was gobsmacked. Nineteen days was a hell of a long time. "I'm thinking it might have to be three months or so," I continued. "I just don't seem to want to stop, once I start drinking. Well, sometimes I do, but usually it's just a freaking nightmare. I'm so sick of not remembering stuff and feeling like such a loser the next day. I'm sick of humiliating myself, and arguing with Dom."

"Oh. But not *forever*?"

"Well, we'll see. I've been reading all these blogs, and people write about the same things that I've experienced, and they think the only way is to stop completely. For good."

"Oh," she repeated. Her eyes were like saucers. I totally understood; the whole concept of forever was blowing my mind too. I held my breath, waiting for her to say something. *Anything.*

Just then, the waiter arrived and placed our meals on the table. Sophie kept her eyes locked on me.

"Well," she said finally. "How are you going to break *that* to your family? Good *luck!*" she burst out laughing, before biting into her sandwich. She knew that my family were big drinkers, and that I was usually the ringleader. It was a role we'd all grown very comfortable with over the years.

*Oh bless you so much for shining a light on the funny side,* I thought. *This is why I love you.*

"God knows!" I giggled with her, feeling the tension melt from my body.

*See? It's not all doom and gloom,* I told myself. *I just need*

*to keep my sense of humour intact and things might actually*
*be okay, after all. Surely.*

~

The very next day, I had plans to meet my ex-colleagues
for drinks. One of them, Chris, had accepted a position in
Europe, and the team were heading to a bar to help him
celebrate. Coincidentally, the very same bar that hosted
Mark and Brooke's wedding reception twelve days earlier.

Jenna texted me, "You have to come, chickie! Everyone
misses you and they're dying to catch up!"

I wanted to go. I missed them too. But I'd be lying
if I said I felt confident about the whole thing. Old Bex
would have been counting down the minutes until it started. New Bex was worried. Everyone knew me as the girl
with the champagne glass in her hand. What the hell was
I going to say to everyone? Not to mention, the last time I
was in that bar, it was pure torture. But I couldn't give up.
What was I going to do, live under a rock for the rest of
my life? All the socialising I was familiar with took place in
bars. I figured I'd better get used to it.

That morning, in preparation, I reviewed my sober
tools. I reminded myself how far I'd come and how important it was to keep going. I visualised feeling proud of
myself when I got home that night, and how amazing I'd
feel the next day.

I thought about *The Sparkle Project* and all the private
coaching I'd done up until that point. When I'd embarked

on a vegan lifestyle, the thought of never eating cheese again filled me with dread. So I made a list of ten things better than cheese, like better digestion, and fewer eczema breakouts. Shifting my focus to what I was gaining, rather than what I was giving up, helped me to feel empowered. Within thirty days, my tastebuds changed, my mantra worked, and I was free. *Damn*, that felt good.

I figured if it had worked to liberate me once, it could work again. I opened my journal to a fresh page and wrote: *10 Things Better Than Wine.*

The blank page stared back, taunting me. *Go on, then.*

I tapped my pen against the page, racking my brain. What was better than wine? I started brainstorming, writing a list of things like:

*Productive mornings. Glowing skin and eyes that sparkle. Better digestion. The smell of fresh, clean sheets beneath my clear and happy head as I fall sleep.*

Determined to reprogram my brain, I flipped to the next page and wrote: *All the Stupid Shit I Haven't Done for the Past Three Weeks.*

I took a deep breath and unleashed it all onto the page. The hangovers. The dread, shame, and paranoia. The lost belongings, memories, and dignity. Damaged relationships. My loss of self.

*Holy crap.* That was a tall price to pay for something that was meant to be 'fun'. My life was so much more peaceful without all of that. I had to see this thing through to the three month mark. I'd be stupid not to.

Still nervous as hell, I headed in to the city and made

a detour to my favourite active wear store. I figured a cute new yoga top would help to cement this new lifestyle into my brain somehow. Plus, I'd have a treat with me as I entered the bar, and all night, I could sneak glimpses at the glossy pink bag and remind myself of the woman I wanted to be. It would be my good luck charm.

I dawdled in the store, taking my sweet time to select a top. It was still early, and I wanted to arrive twenty minutes or so after everyone else got there. There was no way I wanted to be found sitting alone in the hottest new bar in town, nursing a soft drink. *No freaking way.*

Finally, after one last check of the clock, I made my purchase and gathered up the courage to head over. As I walked the couple of blocks to the bar, I thought about all the work drinks I'd been to since I moved back to Perth. How we jokingly referred to midweek drinks as 'Plot Loss Tuesdays' because we'd all go out for *just one drink,* but somehow, they always ended up being the messiest nights of all. Those midweek hangovers were insane.

*And that's why I don't do that shit anymore,* I told myself sternly as I entered the bar, tightly clutching my new purchase.

I spotted my old team crowded around one of the long tables near the entrance. Chris noticed me first and waved me over. When the others saw me, they greeted me with so much warmth and enthusiasm, I temporarily forgot about my nerves.

"Bex! It's so good to see you!" they chorused as they hugged me hello, and I was so glad I'd come. But, of course, the night had only just begun.

"What'll it be?" asked Sean.

"Soda water with fresh lime, please," I chirped, just like I'd practiced.

"Vodka, lime and soda, coming right up!" he sang with a smile, and took off for the bar.

"No, no vodka!" I shouted after him. He turned around. "I'm not drinking. I… I'm on a health kick." I explained, feeling my cheeks burn with the intensity of a supernova. Why oh *why* did my body insist on betraying me?

"Oh," he said, looking confused. "Okay."

"What! A health kick? For how long?" Donna demanded, as Sean made his way to the bar.

"Well. For three months at least," I mumbled.

Jenna gasped. "Are you sure, chickie?" She stared at me, her jaw dropping lower by the second.

"Three months with no alcohol?" said Donna. "Are you *insane*? God, I'd rather go without *food* for three months, than alcohol!" I managed a nervous laugh. I realised that was the very same reaction I would've had just a few short weeks earlier.

"Well, I for one, think you've never looked happier or healthier," Chris came to my rescue. "Cheers!" he said, as Sean handed me my drink, and everyone raised their glasses.

I slurped my first sip, then relaxed a little as the conversation moved on to other topics. I'd forgotten how funny these guys were. Before long, I found myself howling with laughter and forgetting all about my self consciousness. They were so entertaining, and the mood so jovial, that despite my intentions of leaving after two short hours, I stayed for four.

"No! No! Don't go!" they wailed, as I finally made my move. But for the first time in my life, I knew when to call it a night.

As I walked out into the cool night air, I called Dom.

"How was it?" he asked, picking up on the first ring.

"Oh my goodness, I did it! And it was so much fun!" I laughed, delighted to discover that I, Rebecca Weller, could finally socialise sober.

I was still grinning the entire way home. And I was absolutely not even going to *think* about the real test I'd be facing the following weekend.

~

I'd always loved going on holiday with my family. Holidays in general were always a great excuse to drink. *What's that? It's only 11am? Oh well, we're on holiday! Cheers!*

My Mum and Step-Dad had married on a beautiful Autumn day, a week shy of my nineteenth birthday. For the past twenty years, our holidays had been champagne and cocktail celebrations. We didn't know any other kind.

I loved the sweet anticipation in the days leading up to our trips. I loved choosing the crate of champagne to take with us. I loved that my family loved to drink.

Naturally, combining family and alcohol often led to an argument or two. And usually by about the third day, I felt sick, tired, and grumpy, but I put all of that aside. In my mind, drinking—especially for many days in a row—was always fun and exciting.

This year, Mum had hired a beautiful beach house for an Easter family getaway. And all I could think was, *I'm not at 30 days yet. I'm still on such shaky ground.*

On Friday afternoon, as Dom and I drove up the coast, the butterflies threw a party inside my rib cage. I didn't think my family would give me a hard time, exactly, but I suspected it would be strange and awkward. I remembered the handful of times in the past when one of them hadn't wanted to drink—usually because they were feeling ill from the day before—and what a fuss I'd made. There were very few hangovers that stopped me from drinking the next day and wanting everyone around me to get involved. I wouldn't take no for an answer.

The shoe was well and truly on the other foot now, and I hoped they'd be more understanding and gracious than I ever was.

The house was gorgeous. Double-storey, with polished wooden floors and colourful pieces of art hanging throughout.

"Cocktail?" my sister asked, after we'd all hugged hello and moved to the kitchen.

"Uh, no thanks. I've brought mocktail ingredients," I stammered, awkward as ever.

"Oh." She placed a bottle of vodka back down on the kitchen bench. "Are you not drinking at *all*? But I read your blog post about 'ten things better than wine'. So it's only wine that's a bitch," she joked. "You can still drink vodka!"

The butterflies dive-bombed into my stomach, making me nauseous. "No, I... I'm taking a break from all of it," I mumbled, attempting to avoid eye contact.

"Oh," she said, looking disappointed. "Well, that's no fun!"

"I can still be fun without alcohol," I protested.

"Can you?" she asked, raising an eyebrow.

*If only I knew.*

As she carried her drink out to the deck, I worried about what she thought of me. I worried that I'd be left out. I worried a lot.

I pulled ginger lemonade ingredients from our cooler bag, frustrated to find myself once again fighting back tears. Desperately, I reminded myself how close I was to thirty days. If I was getting this upset, and it was this hard for me to go without alcohol, what further proof did I need that I was addicted and actually needed to do this?

*They'll still love you, no matter what's in your glass*, I reassured myself, trying to hold it together.

The afternoon dragged. Even though I knew I was doing the best thing for me, and Dom was an angel drinking mocktails in solidarity, I couldn't help but feel envious that my family were drinking. I was sure that the afternoon felt awkward for everyone, and my sobriety was the cause of it.

I used to be one of those people who could just laugh things off. I missed carefree, fun Bex who could always hide her feelings behind her glass. All this reality and raw emotion, *all the freaking time*, was driving me nuts. I tried to focus on how lovely it was to be staying in the beautiful beach house, but deep down, I felt miserable. No-one had ever accused me of being a party pooper, but I felt like one now, and I didn't like it one little bit.

Late in the afternoon, I went to the kitchen cupboard to find some more snacks. If I couldn't drink, I was jolly well going to gorge myself on junk food. As I reached up to grab a packet of chips, I spied a wine bottle towards the back. An open bottle of red, most likely belonging to my parents.

*Well, look at that*, grinned the beast, saliva dripping from his lips. *Just pour yourself a quick glass. Everyone else is still outside. No-one will see you. No-one ever has to know.*

Shaking, I closed the cupboard door and backed away.

~

The next morning dawned sunny and bright, and I felt elated. I'd achieved another huge milestone; sober for an entire night on a family holiday.

I hummed as I dressed. This self-trust business felt more delicious than I'd ever imagined. Not to mention, *hallelujah*, no hangover.

Granted, Dom and I had gone to bed at 9pm while my family stayed up until the early hours, but *still*. I'd stuck to my guns and lived to tell the tale, and for now, that was the most important thing.

When I headed downstairs for breakfast, I found my

parents and sister sitting at the dining table, looking a little worse for wear. I doubted they'd be up for much partying that night, and for that I was thankful. It meant my sobriety wouldn't feel as weird.

*Note to self: the first night of any holiday will be the biggest party night. Arrive on the second day.*

The next two days felt very different. Partly because I relaxed into my non-drinking identity a little more, and partly because, with the first excited night out of their systems, my family's drinking died down too. We chatted, went for walks on the beach, visited local markets, and shared deep belly laughs.

On the final morning of our stay, sunbeams streamed through the wooden blinds, gently waking me. Dom was still sleeping peacefully beside me. I stretched and smiled as I realised what this day meant. *Oh, the incredible magnitude of it all.*

I reached for my phone and checked my trusty little tracker app, just to be sure. Yep, thirty days. *Thirty whole days.* It seemed impossible, and yet it was true. I let the moment sink in, my mind whirling. One whole month alcohol-free. No sneaking a sip here or there, like the times I'd attempted sobriety before. This was thirty days of pure, full, complete sobriety.

My family were staying another night, but Dom and I decided to go back to the city that day.

"Come on, it's your birthday. Just stay!" my family pleaded as we packed up the car. But I knew I wouldn't want to watch them drinking that night. It was Day 30, it was the last birthday of my thirties, and I just wanted to go home. I wanted to celebrate in a new way, and show myself exactly how I planned to look after myself in future.

As we pulled out of the driveway and waved goodbye, I couldn't help feeling sad that I was leaving them. But at the same time, I felt proud of myself for finding the courage to make my wellbeing a priority.

"You did it, sweetie! Happy birthday," Dom smiled, as he drove us home.

I smiled back at him. My body tingled with emotions, but mostly, I felt calm. In my head, I tried to name the other emotions. It was a game I'd been playing to help make sense of the hot mess of feelings inside me for the past month. Two words bubbled up. *Peaceful. Content.* I was getting better at this.

When we arrived home, for the first time in my adult life, I celebrated my birthday sober. Instead of my usual cocktails, champagne, and dancing-on-tables celebration, I spent the night cuddling with Dom on the couch. We made fajitas for dinner—my favourite—and shared some fancy raw chocolate for dessert. I filled my crystal goblet with sparkling mineral water and fresh lime juice, and we watched an '80s flick.

It felt really good. Wholesome. Healthy. *Right.* It felt every bit the delicious milestone.

Suddenly, in a blinding flash of inspiration, it occurred to me. *Maybe I've been approaching this entire experiment all wrong.*

# NINE

During breakfast the next morning, I mulled it over. *What if everything I ever believed about my idea of fun, was wrong?* Could it be that I got so drunk at events because I wasn't comfortable there in the first place?

I looked across the table at Dom. I'd actually *loved* celebrating my birthday in such a chilled-out way. Maybe—just maybe—instead of trying to fit myself into an old mould, what I needed was to embrace a complete *reinvention*. I tapped my spoon against my forehead. *But how?*

"We should get fit," I announced.

"Okay…" Dom said, looking up with amusement from the article he was reading.

"Exercise gets the endorphins pumping, right? It'll give me the highs that booze gave me, but without all the nasty stuff. Plus, it'll help me deal with stress and emotions. *And*, we'll sleep better."

Dom grinned. "Okedokey. I always want to exercise more, but you never seem that keen on it." He was right. Despite turning my life upside down to become a health coach, I'd never fallen in love with exercise.

"Well, I'm different now. Things are different," I told him. Meaning, *now that I was breaking up with alcohol, exercise seemed like the perfect new obsession.*

For years, I'd loved organising social events, my friends often calling me their 'Social Organiser' or 'Clipboard Queen'. It was a role I missed terribly, and I realised how empty I felt without it. If I wasn't the woman always first in line at the bar, ordering champagne for everyone and helping them have a good time, *who was I?* There were still two months left of this challenge, and I was determined to get rid of this gnawing feeling, *pronto*.

All fired up, I opened my laptop and jumped online to search for new things to try. Okay, so our usual cocktail events were out, but surely this was a great chance to try new things as a group.

I clicked around until I found a few classes that sounded exciting; a sexy dance class, yoga in the park, and aerial pilates. Brimming with enthusiasm, I emailed the dates and details to our group of friends.

"Job done!" I told Dom. "I've invited everyone and it can be a whole new chapter for us all."

"Mhm," he smiled, giving me a doubtful look that I chose to ignore. This was a great idea, he'd see.

It'd always been easy to get our group excited about going to a bar or gig, but as the hours turned into days, there appeared to be a lack of enthusiasm for this new master plan of mine. As the polite 'no, thank you' responses continued to trickle in, I grew more and more worried.

The beast had a field day. *Keep this up and you're going to be a sad loser sitting at home by yourself, while the rest of the world is out living their exciting, glamorous lives.*

I didn't want to believe it. I didn't want to quit this sobriety experiment, but the thought of spending another night standing in a pub with only soda water in my glass was awful.

In desperation, I racked my brain for a Plan B. I'd always encouraged my clients to take responsibility for their own lives; to jump firmly into the drivers seat and change anything they didn't like. Well, I didn't like going to the same old places, doing the same old things, and expecting different results. Nope, if I was going to embrace this challenge whole-heartedly, I was going to have to do things I'd never done before. And one of those things was to nurture friendships with people who didn't drink.

I pulled out my day planner and noted a few time slots that looked good over the coming weeks. My schedule was tight, due to our mad entrepreneurial workload, but I was a woman on a mission. With a few dates in mind, I texted my health coach friends, Holly, Diana and Zara, and suggested brunches, yoga classes, and walks around the river.

And then I waited. I stared at my phone, willing it to beep with positive replies. If this plan didn't work, I was fresh out of options, and the thought was too depressing to bear.

Finally, I heard my phone beep. Then beep again. I held my breath as I read the replies, and almost burst with happiness. Before I knew it, I had a bunch of healthy dates to look forward to.

As I closed my diary, I felt empowered. *Excited*, even. Month one of this experiment had been incredibly challenging, with my first sober wedding, work function, family holiday, and birthday.

*Month two is going to be a whole lot different*, I assured myself.

~

The following morning as I got dressed, I visualised the woman I wanted to be. The fact was, I could throw as many pity parties as I wanted, but no-one was coming to do this work for me. I was in control, I had the power to change, and it was up to me to create my new life.

Never one to do things by halves, I resolved to launch myself straight into the next phase.

"I'm doing a spring clean!" I yelled out to Dom, pulling clothes and shoes from our wardrobe like a maniac. Never mind that it was autumn, or that I was meant to be working. This was suddenly the most urgent task in the world.

When it came to my belongings, I'd always displayed a

deep sentimentality that could easily be mistaken for unhealthy attachment. Now, all this *stuff* felt stifling. I craved
a clear out.

"Okedokey," he called back, leaving me to continue
with whatever crazy plan I was up to now.

The plan was Minimalist. I wasn't deluded enough to
think that I'd get there right away, but I was desperate to
do something—anything—to make myself feel better. I
needed to escape from all this emotion. I needed to get out
of my head for a while.

Plus, it felt symbolic somehow. Like I was shedding
the old me. It had been six weeks. Six weeks of relentless
flashbacks and unwelcome memories of all the ways I'd let
people down. And most of all, how I'd let myself down. I
didn't want to be that clueless, immature, lost woman anymore. I wasn't sure how long I planned to stick to complete sobriety, but I knew I didn't want to go back *there*
ever again.

I spent hours frantically clearing and sorting. I filled
two huge plastic bags on the bed; one to donate and one
to throw away. When I finished with the wardrobe, I started on my jewellery box. Then the study. Then the kitchen.

I was a woman possessed.

"Shall we make some dinner?" Dom asked eventually,
and I looked up to realise it was getting dark outside. I'd
spent the entire day decluttering.

"Sure," I said. "Would you help me take these bags
down to the car first?"

It took us four trips. But rather than feeling sad about

kissing my things goodbye, I felt deliriously light and happy. It felt like freedom.

The following week, I met Diana for brunch at Solomon's Café. We thought about trying somewhere new, but their food was just too scrumptious to resist. "Let's sit at a different table, at least," I laughed, when I met her out front.

We chose a cozy table near the barista station; the heavenly smell of coffee making me second-guess my juice order.

"How's the not-drinking thing going?" Diana asked, taking a sip of her carrot and turmeric juice.

For a second, I considered being blasé about it; smiling and waving it off, like it was nothing. Sophie's voice popped into my head like she was Obi-Wan Kenobi to my Luke Skywalker, "Even when you're really drunk, Bex, you're very guarded."

Suddenly it occurred to me; how much I'd always craved intimacy, while also being afraid of it. Like if I opened myself up just a crack, all the deepest, darkest parts of me would come tumbling out and I'd never be able to shove them back in again.

As I looked into the warmth of Diana's eyes, I knew I wanted to get better at opening up. I longed for more truth in my life.

"Well," I said, taking a deep breath. "Honestly? The best way I could describe it, is it feels like heartbreak. Like a break up. I swear I've cried more in the past two months than I have in my entire life. I've cried because I missed it. I've cried because I couldn't imagine the rest of my life without it. I felt devastated that something so stupid could have such an incredible hold over me. And sometimes seeing other people drinking feels exactly like seeing an ex-boyfriend, and all the emotions come flooding back."

She nodded, waiting for me to continue.

"But it's getting easier. I guess like any breakup; you cry, you avoid them, and then you start rebuilding your life. It's been almost two months now, and it does get easier every day. Some days actually feel amazing, like I escaped an abusive relationship and am free to start again. Usually the days when I'm taking great care of myself. Of course, stress doesn't help, but that's a bit tricky to avoid when you're running your own biz, huh?" I smiled, knowing she'd understand exactly what I meant.

"Absolutely," she laughed.

Two months earlier, IIN had hired me to provide business mentoring to their Australian health coaching students. I was thrilled and honoured to be offered such a role, and I tried not to think about the extra workload. My schedule was already intense, with running *The Sparkle Project* and doing all the usual new biz stuff. Marketing, accounting, legal, blogging, newsletters, social media, building referral networks, discussing revenue streams, and generally floundering about, hoping like crazy we'll be able to make it all work.

As Diana told me about her latest business adventures,

I realised how blessed I was to have the love and support of other health coaches. To be forming close bonds with other people who were doing similar things, and who totally 'got' it.

The part of me that loved clinging to my old identity loosened her grip, just a little bit.

~

The following week, Holly invited me over to her place for an all-day brainstorming session. We were both keen to create beautiful membership sites for our clients, and as it was something neither of us had done it before, we thought it'd be fun to figure it out together.

I arrived to find her already sitting at her computer. She'd moved her desk into the centre of the living room and had set up another table up next to it, creating a makeshift desk for me. She'd lined the desks with pretty notepapers, coloured pens, and sachets of herbal tea. As I took in the scene, I felt choked with emotion. It looked like the beauty and innocence of childhood friendship.

Noticing the tears in my eyes, she hugged me.

As instructed, I'd brought my laptop, so we fired it up, and got to work. We had a blast. Sitting side-by-side, sipping endless cups of herbal tea, and giggling whenever we hit a technical roadblock. We stopped only for as long as it took to eat the delicious chickpea curry Holly had made us for lunch.

Later, as I drove home, a contented, blissful feeling

came over me—something I rarely felt. I sang along to the tunes on the radio. It was Day 60, and I was forming strong new friendships, and learning new things every day. I knew it might all feel different tomorrow, but for now at least, life felt amazing.

# TEN

My euphoria didn't last long. By the time Friday rolled around, I was furious. Furious with the people drinking in the bar we walked past at lunchtime, with our huge workload, and with this whole challenge.

I'd read a blog post once by a woman who'd received what she deemed a 'sign from the Universe' to remain sober. In truth, I felt like I'd seen a big neon sign to stop drinking at the Earth Angel event. But often, I wondered if the Universe would send me a sign that my life would be permanently better without alcohol.

That Friday, I found out.

Dom and I were waiting to catch the central transit bus

home from the city. The shiny display on my phone told me it was 3pm, and I realised I'd foolishly skipped lunch. I was cold, hungry and tired. It was just one of those days where nothing seems to go right.

"What's the *matter*?" Dom asked. I hadn't spoken to him since he told me I couldn't buy a cute top I saw on sale. He was worried about our cash flow. I knew he was right, but that only made it all the more frustrating.

*What's the matter?* I fumed in my head. *Oh, who the hell knows! I'm feeling emotions faster than I can identify them and the whole experience is nauseating and exhausting. It's like a sick rollercoaster that never ends, no matter how much I beg and plead for it to stop. I'm sick of sobriety, but most of all, I'm sick of myself.*

But I didn't say that. I said, "Well, what's the point in *living*? I can't have any time off, I can't buy a new top, I can't eat junk food, and I can't drink!" *Hello!* The beast was awake, my inner brat was spinning out of control, and I couldn't do a damned thing about it.

The bus arrived, no doubt to Dom's great relief. I clambered on board, fighting back tears. I found us a seat, and plonked myself down in a sulk, furious with anything and everything. I *dared* the stupid Universe to send me a sign that I shouldn't just crack open a bottle of wine the second I got home. The bus took off with an awful jolt that only amplified my state.

At the next stop, a woman stumbled onto the bus, and slumped into the seat directly in front of ours. Her hair and clothes were a mess, and she smelt awful. As the bus drove off again, I saw her raise a small bottle of whiskey to her lips and take a giant swig.

I felt like the wind had been knocked out of me. As I struggled to breathe, blood pounded through my head, deafening me. I couldn't look away. Glug after glug, she worked her way through the bottle, stopping only to yell out incoherently to the driver.

A couple of stops later—one stop before ours—she staggered off the bus.

As Dom and I stood to alight, I was shaking. The bus had barely pulled away before I had a meltdown. "Why aren't you sick of me?" I demanded, tears streaming down my cheeks. "*I'm* sick of me!"

In the middle of the street, he pulled me into a hug, and I sobbed for what felt like an eternity.

As we finally turned and walked back to our apartment, my inner brat counted her blessings. *Message received, Universe. Loud and clear.*

~

Our workload over the next couple of weeks saw no reprieve. I was proud of Dom and I for finding the courage to follow our passions—especially at the same time—but it was all so new and scary as well. As stressful and hectic as it was, most days I gratefully sank into it. Work provided a welcome distraction from the avalanche of emotions and memories that insisted on crashing down on my head.

One morning, try as I might, I couldn't ignore the

growing anxiety gnawing away inside me. "Okay, fine!" I said out loud to my insides, putting my pen down with a sigh. "You have my attention. What is it?"

"Did you say something?" Dom said, appearing in the study doorway.

"Oh I'm just talking to myself," I said, with a wry smile. "First sign of madness."

As he smiled at me, something clicked. "You know what it is?" I said. "I'm scared of emotions. It's like I've been running from them all my life. And now they're coming for me. It's payback time."

I thought about all the ways I'd been able to avoid my emotions in the past. How often and completely I'd drowned them. Creating drama, scrolling through social media, shopping, and binge-watching television shows. And most of all, how I'd drunk myself into oblivion.

What if 'controlling my drinking' didn't mean learning how to moderate, but creating a life so complete and fulfilling that alcohol couldn't add anything I didn't already have? Is that what this was all about? Did I need to create a life—and a relationship with myself—that I didn't want to escape from?

I sighed deeply. All this navel gazing was exhausting. Where the hell was that Day 60 reprieve I'd been promised?

As the day rolled on, it only got worse. "Oh, for God's sake!" I wailed, bursting into tears when the pasta sauce jar I was trying to open went flying out of my hands and smashed across the entire kitchen floor.

"Sweetie, it's okay. Let me help you," Dom said, grabbing the paper towels.

His kindness only made me sob even harder. I felt like a pathetic excuse for a human being. I couldn't even make dinner without falling apart.

"Go and sit down," he said. "It's okay."

I traipsed to the study and collapsed into my chair. This was getting ridiculous. What could I do to make myself feel better? My head and body ached with the intensity of it all. I wished I owned one of those incredible full-body massage chairs they had at the hairdresser.

*Bingo,* I thought, reaching for my phone.

~

"Your hair actually feels a lot thicker since you started eating healthier," my hairdresser said, as we chatted about the recipes on my *Vegan Sparkles* blog.

"Does it?" I asked, surprised and delighted. All my life I'd wished for thicker hair.

"And you have quite a sweet tooth, don't you," she said.

"Oh," I laughed. "I suppose I do. But nothing like I used to".

Suddenly I had a blinding flashback of the rock bottom of my sugar addiction. I was twenty-three years old and had begged my then-boyfriend to stop on our way home so I could buy a chocolate bar. Inside the store, I quickly grabbed three bars and made for the register.

"What!" he exclaimed as he tried to grab them from

my hands. "*One*, not three. Put them back."

"No!" I hissed, clinging to them for dear life. Seeing the look on my face—and no doubt wanting to avoid a scene—he let go. Filled with shame, I fought back tears as we made our way through the checkout. I felt completely out of control.

As the blowdryer swirled warm air around my face, my mind went into overdrive. I'd read countless articles about sugar stimulating the same reward centre in the brain as alcohol. So potentially, all the tools I'd used to overcome my sugar addiction should help me to overcome my alcohol issues too, right? A blog post was brewing and I couldn't wait to get back to my computer.

The minute I got home, I cracked open my laptop and started typing: *10 Ways to Conquer Your Sugar Cravings.*

In the blog post, I shared every tool I'd used, including drinking more water, minimising caffeine, eating sweet vegetables, whole fruit and healthy fats, getting more exercise, and even EFT.

As I hit 'publish' and closed my laptop, I realised how many of these healthy habits I'd strayed from. I'd managed to avoid refined sugar for years, but over the past couple of months, I'd been hitting it hard in an attempt to soothe myself. I knew I wasn't doing myself any favours. I understood exactly how sugar impacted the body and wreaked havoc on the brain, skin, and hormones. Not to mention, on energy levels, and the central nervous system. For the sake of my emotions and sanity, I committed to getting back on track.

I thought about the question Dom asked me when I first told him about the beast. *What are you really craving?* Deep down, I knew it wasn't actually the alcohol itself. So what was it? That feeling of letting loose; of wild abandon? Or the sense of connection I thought I got when I drank with people? Was I really craving more fun, adventure, affection, and freedom in my life?

I'd always believed I loved drinking because it was 'fun'. Had I really been drinking to fill an emptiness inside?

~

"I think they're planning to go somewhere for drinks afterwards," Dom said as we dressed for his friend Ben's wedding ceremony. This was the first of two weddings Ben and Alana had planned. It was to be held at a registrar office in the city; a mere formality so that they could head off on their global travels for the next few months as a married couple. Their huge, official wedding party was scheduled for later in the year.

I wished the mention of heading out for drinks didn't make me nervous, but it did. It had been exactly ninety days. I felt more comfortable in my sobriety every day, but celebrating this milestone by heading to a wedding party, well, it just felt like tempting fate.

The registrar office was beautiful. We'd been there before for another friend's ceremony, and it was all plush carpeting, elegant wall trimmings, and sweeping river views. The bride and groom had invited about thirty of their closest friends and family, and everyone was dressed up and in a celebratory mood.

"Okay, everyone can come through now," the celebrant said, waving us all into a more formal room.

Cameras flashed as the couple took their places at the front of the room. The hushed silence was laced with anticipation.

As Ben and Alana stared into each others eyes, I found myself feeling choked with emotion. Three months earlier, I would have been here, but not *here*. I knew without a doubt that the majority of my mind would have been firmly fixed in a countdown to the first drink.

If there was one thing I'd discovered over the past few weeks, it was that allowing myself to be open and vulnerable was confronting and painful. Tuning in meant coming face-to-face with memories and emotions I didn't want to deal with. But there was something even scarier; imagining a life half-lived. By closing myself off from pain, I saw that I'd also cut myself off from all the beauty and magic of greater intuition, creativity, depth, growth, and love.

Now, I felt completely present and in awe, witnessing a moment of pure love. Despite feeling embarrassed about the tears in my eyes, it felt incredible.

"Congratulations!" the crowd cheered as the ceremony concluded, and we spilled out into the reception area.

"We're heading to The Royal," Ben said to us. "You guys are coming, right?"

"Of course," Dom said. My stomach dropped. The Royal was the waterfront venue where I'd drunk myself silly in the middle of the day with Rosie. The Universe seemed determined to not only send me a message, but to underline it with a huge, permanent marker.

"You okay?" Dom asked, noticing the serious look on my face, after Ben had moved on to talk to other guests.

"Yeah," I breathed, managing a weak smile. He smiled back, taking my hand in his and giving it a reassuring squeeze.

Half of the guests headed down to the carpark. The bar was a little too far to walk to in heels, but not far enough to bother calling a cab, so we followed the other guests down to the central transit bus. On the way, we continued to make polite small talk, answering the inevitable question, "So how do you know the bride and groom?"

At the bar, Ben's brother had organised a large private section for the wedding party. I was relieved to find that it was inside, and not in the alfresco area where I'd sat with Rosie.

"Shall I get us some drinks?" Dom asked, and I nodded. As he disappeared towards the bar, I looked around for someone to talk to. *Life Of The Party to Awkward Mute in just three months*, I joked to myself. It felt like the first day of school. Taking a deep breath, I shyly approached a group, hoping they'd invite me into their conversation. Ben's mum and two sisters joined the group a moment after I did.

"Hey Bex, Ben told me you have a vegan blog. That's so cool!" one of his sisters said. "Is it hard being vegan?"

*Not as hard as being newly sober*, I thought, before

laughing and relaxing into the conversation. I was over-joyed to discover that they were all lovely. Warm, kind and wildly entertaining, just like Ben. They were drinking co-lourful, delicious-looking cocktails and I tried not to feel too envious as Dom returned to hand me a sparkling min-eral water.

*Tomorrow you'll be glad*, I reminded myself. *Ninety days is not a hundred days, and you said a hundred.*

The wedding party grew more animated as the hours rolled on. More people poured into the bar, fresh from work and ready to celebrate the start of the weekend, and the bar's ambient volume quickly rose.

Feeling fatigued, I scanned the room for Dom. He caught my eye and raised his chin in a question like, *Ready?*

I nodded and smiled. *God, I love this man.*

He strode over to me, swiftly taking charge like Rhett Butler, or Don Draper on a good day. Together, we made our rounds, saying goodbye. Before I knew it, we were outside.

"Thank you!" I laughed, hugging him with wild relief.

"That's okay," he grinned, "I was ready to leave too. Let's get some dinner. Hungry?"

"Starving!" I beamed and grabbed his hand.

We strolled along the waterfront until we came across a cute little Thai restaurant, complete with gold chairs, ma-genta tablecloths, and twinkling lanterns hanging from the ceiling.

The waitress brought us our coconut waters complete with beautiful orchids decorating the glasses, and I felt overcome with gratitude. I imagined how this night would have played out if it had happened a few months earlier. Weddings had always been a signal to me to go absolutely mad, and you can bet your bottom dollar that this one would have been no exception. I would have made a fool of myself and spent the next few months drowning in shame, dreading seeing all the guests again at the big wedding later in the year.

Instead, I'd left feeling proud of myself. Better yet, I was sitting here, in a pretty restaurant, looking into the eyes of the man I adored. I knew I'd feel amazing as I tucked myself into bed that night, my clear and grateful head hitting the pillow. And that I'd feel even better the next morning.

*Obviously,* the beast whispered, *you don't have a* real *problem. You've been sober for three whole months.*

*That's true,* I thought, as the waitress placed our meals on the table.

*You've proven your point,* the beast grinned, excited to be getting through to me at last. *You* like *alcohol, but you don't* need *it. Now you can drink again like a normal person.*

I took a sip of my coconut juice and wondered if the beast was on to something.

# ELEVEN

As I opened my eyes on the morning of Day 99, an un-welcome thought popped into my head. *If you don't need it anymore, then why do you need it?* I couldn't quite wrap my head around this, so I decided to put it out of my mind entirely.

That afternoon, Louise and Meghan picked me up on the way to Ashleigh's baby shower. I was standing out the front of my building, giddy with excitement about seeing everyone, when Louise pulled up. I quickly jumped in the back, clutching my gift for the baby.

"So are you drinking today, Bex?" Louise asked as she adjusted her rear-view mirror. Meghan swivelled in the front seat so she could look at me.

"No, I think I need a bit longer," I admitted. "I'm feeling so much healthier and happier without it, and I just want to wait and see what happens."

As the cloud around my brain had continued to lift, it occurred to me just how muddled I'd been towards the end of my drinking. Fragments of memories squished together, tangled around snippets of conversations, dreams, and television shows I'd watched while under the influence. The whole hotchpotch was utterly confusing.

Life felt so much more stable now, and I loved waking up every morning feeling fresh and grounded, and one hundred percent *real*. I was beginning to actually trust and like myself, and I didn't want to lose that. Not yet. Hopefully, not ever.

We were one of the last to arrive; the living room already filled with smiling women, balloons, and baby gifts. As we chatted to the other ladies, I felt surprisingly calm and at ease. The usual introductions didn't make me squirm with awkwardness. It didn't bother me that most of the other guests were drinking champagne while I drank sparkling apple juice. I didn't even feel the pressure to carry a conversation. I was so chilled out, I wasn't sure I was even the same person.

Hours later, after the fun and games had subsided, the energy in the room began to dip and people started to leave.

Another friend, Claire, was waiting for her ride home. She nodded towards my glass. "You still not drinking?" she asked.

"Nope," I smiled.

"Oh well, when in Rome," she shrugged, pouring herself another glass of champagne. I knew what she was doing. She was trying to speed up time; make it more fun, get over the boring bits. I'd done it a thousand times myself. Meanwhile, I felt completely relaxed and content to be me. Not chasing more fun, desperate for more excitement, grasping for more booze.

Back when I socialised with a drink in my hand, part of my mind was always preoccupied. *Did I bring enough wine? Will anyone notice if I pour another? What if we run out?* Now, when I spoke to people, I was absolutely focused on what they were saying. Better yet, I remembered everything we talked about, and that sense of honest connection filled me with joy.

I thought I needed to drink to feel confident. And yet, the longer I went without drinking, the more confident I felt in every situation. Life was so incredibly peaceful without all that internal angst and drama.

Later, as Louise drove us home, I marvelled at my mood and what a difference a few weeks makes. As much as I missed drinking, I certainly wasn't in any hurry to rush back to the land of hangovers, shame, and regret. But *forever* still felt too scary, too infinite. Too huge for me to hold my hand on my heart and promise on. For now, all I knew was that sobriety was too beautiful a sanctuary for me to give up anytime soon. I'd worked so hard to get here and this feeling was more sublime than I could have ever imagined.

A thought entered my mind, *Why not six months?*

I smiled. So the Good Wolf was awake. I pursed my lips as I considered the idea. I definitely wasn't ready to commit to a sober Christmas or New Years Eve. Six months would take me into September, and that actually didn't sound too awful.

*Okay*, I declared to myself. *Six months it is.*

~

"Have you started that blog post yet?" Dom asked me for the millionth time.

"No. I mean, should I really bother? Do people really want to hear about it?"

"Yes!" he said, exasperated. "It's an important story. Get to work."

As always, he recognised resistance when he saw it. I'd told him that I wanted to write a blog post about my sobriety journey. After years of hiding my drinking—plotting, scheming and lying about it—I craved honesty. I was sick of secrets. I knew that having public accountability would be good for me, but above all, I wanted to reach out to anyone who was struggling with the same battles and demons. I wanted them to know that they were loved, and they were not alone.

But I was scared. I was supposed to be a health coach, for crying out loud. What if no-one wanted to work with me after I shared this story? What if everyone thought I was just a cork sniff away from complete self-destruction? What if I had to go crawling back to the corporate world, but my reputation was tainted there too and no-one would hire me? What if I really *did* become the homeless alcoholic stereotype? *What if, what if, what if…*

I knew that the majority of this fear lived only in my imagination. And yet, I was terrified. I sat down to write, and promptly burst into tears.

"Oh, hey. What's going on?" Dom asked, coming into the study. "Come here." He pulled me out of the chair and into a bear hug, and I sobbed on his shoulder until I felt a little better.

"All this reality all the time is so freakin' *intense!*" I half-joked, and we both let out a bit of a laugh.

"This is something to be really proud of, sweetie. Don't be ashamed of the struggles you've overcome." I thought of my coaching sessions and all the times I'd said similar things to my clients. *The truth will set you free. Embrace your vulnerability. Own your story, don't let it own you.*

He was right. I remembered how much the sobriety blogs had helped me, and how I'd wished they weren't all anonymous. I sat down at my laptop again. By hook or by crook, I was going to conquer this mountain.

I'd written my previous post, *10 Things Better Than Wine*, in very general terms. This post would be more of a confession; of actually admitting the truth about my past. It was hard to know where to begin.

I started typing, sharing all the reasons I'd wanted to stop drinking in the first place. The anxiety, the shame, the nausea. How I found it so hard to stop drinking once I started. My biggest fears about sobriety; that I might never have fun, or fit in, ever again. And above all, how I craved peace and freedom from this ridiculous, traumatic pattern.

When I was done, I read it back, and was surprised to find that it made sense. With a trembling finger, I clicked 'publish'. My heart raced. I felt hot and cold at the same time, dizzy, nauseous, and exposed. My first blog post about sobriety, *100 Days Without a Drink - Part 1*, was live.

Within minutes, comments and emails started flooding in. Beautiful messages full of warmth, love and compassion, like:

> *"Well done, Bex! You should be very proud! A true soul searching experience for you, one that will be life changing and so fulfilling. Not an easy thing to post out there for the world to see, so I commend you on your strength, courage and determination! Thanks for your inspiration, you're amazing."*

> *"So beautifully written and I can definitely relate. For me it was also so very difficult to give up the party but I'm so glad my boozy life is behind me. Here's to a bright sparkling future for all of us who make the toughest choices and emerge from the other side with renewed joy. Thank you for sharing."*

> *"I just wanted to drop you a note thanking you for all that you do. This post really hit home with me. I re-*

*ally want to start thinking about why I am drinking, and more specifically why I have more than one glass (or bottle)! Should be an interesting learning process. Thanks again. You're amazing!"*

One week later, my head was still spinning. I was so relieved to know I wasn't going to lose my clients and readers by being honest. It was all out on the table now. No hiding, no running. I finally knew the meaning of the word authentic.

As I whizzed up a green smoothie for breakfast, I pondered the bigger picture. What would I be capable of if I stayed true to this path; embracing sobriety, maturity, responsibility, and all those things I'd previously shunned? I could already see how much this experiment was transforming my relationships. As if people could sense that I trusted myself more, which in turn, made them trust me more.

As I sat down to write part two of my *100 Days Without a Drink* blog series, I felt much braver.

This time, I shared some of the tools I'd used to get through the first thirty days. Things like my favourite lists, forums, books, blogs, and apps, and how I'd committed to a one hundred day challenge. I also shared an insight into just how challenging the first thirty days had been.

Again, the messages and emails flooded in, astounding me with their outpouring of love and support, and the depth of suffering that was going on behind closed doors:

*"I feel like you are talking about me! I have also just ordered the book, written the list, and signed up to the forums you mentioned. Thank you so much for sharing this, it has come at the perfect time for me."*

*"Thank you for inspiring me to take a break from the booze. I'm on Day 10 and learning a lot from this time. Can't wait to hear more from you!"*

*"This is really amazing. You have inspired me to try something similar. I've gone 5 days (back in January), and that's the most for, gosh, more than ten years. It's otherwise been daily. I look forward to reading more of your story!"*

*"Thanks for the inspiration, Bec. It's Day 3, and after a really crappy work day, which would usually mean a bottle of Sauv Blanc to dull the stress, I went to the shops instead and came home and enjoyed a mineral water. Gave myself a pat on the back! I have been battling with my love of wine getting out of hand for a while now. Your blog really hit home and spurred me on. Next big step: an alcohol-free weekend! 100 days here I come. Thank you!"*

As I read through the messages, my heart overflowing, a new email appeared my inbox.

*Subject: Sunday Times Magazine enquiry*

*Hi Bex,*
*I'm writing a story for STM on the change in body focus from thin to fit and healthy.*
*I would love to interview you for this feature article. Are you interested?*

*Was I interested?* I read and re-read the email to make sure I wasn't imagining it. *The Sunday Times Magazine?*

"Dom!" I bellowed from the study.

"What is it?" he tumbled through the doorway, looking worried.

"Read this!" I jumped out of my office chair so he could confirm I wasn't hallucinating.

"Cool!" he laughed. "Write back! Tell her yes."

My mind couldn't quite process it, but I wrote back and we set up a time for a phone interview.

Later that day, the journalist called. Her questions were brilliant, and thankfully I forgot my nerves as soon as I started talking. I spoke about self-love being the real key to health and happiness, and I just hoped the article would reflect this, and be free of any aspect of body shaming. The journalist seemed lovely, but it was my first experience with mainstream media, and I was apprehensive.

As I hung up the phone, Dom reappeared in the doorway. "She asked if their photographer could come and take a photo of me next week," I told him, dumbfounded.

"That's fantastic! You're amazing, my little health coach," he smiled and pulled me into a hug.

STM. *Wow.* I remembered the photo shoot I did during a trip to Sydney the previous year. I'd booked a photographer to take some headshots for my website. Feeling nervous the night before the shoot, I got stuck into the vino, even though I swore I wouldn't. The next day I felt ridiculous; red-eyed and hungover at a photo shoot for my wellness website.

At least I wouldn't have to worry about hangovers this time. No sleeping past my alarm, no waking up in last night's outfit, no worrying about whether the smell of alcohol was seeping out of my pores.

There was another worry niggling away at me, though; that stepping into the spotlight might bring more readers to my blog. Which meant more people might see my posts about sobriety. Was I ready for that?

~

The following Sunday, Dom and I were up early. We were due to visit my family, and we'd been up late the night before, desperately trying to fix something on my website. We were determined to resolve it before we had to leave.

Hours later, we still weren't any closer to fixing the damn thing.

Temporarily defeated, we walked to our local café seeking the solace of a quick cappuccino break. Completely stressed out, I didn't hear my phone when it buzzed the first time.

"I think that's your phone," Dom said, as it buzzed for the second time. I reached into my bag to retrieve it. It was a text message from a family friend I hadn't spoken to in months. *That's odd*, I thought, opening the message. A split-second later, a photo appeared on the screen. It was my picture in the Sunday Times Magazine, along with the message, "We are so proud!"

I gasped and held my phone out for Dom to see. He laughed and jumped out of his seat, calling out to the waiter to ask if they had a copy. The waiter shrugged. Apparently they didn't receive their usual delivery that day.

"Oh well," Dom grinned. "Your family will have a copy. We'll read it when we get there."

Thrilled to receive good news after one hell of a morning, we guzzled our coffees and jumped straight into the car.

My family had the magazine open on the kitchen bench when we arrived, and I smiled, dizzy with bliss, as I read the three-page feature that included interviews with two other Perth wellness babes. The article was titled, *Meet the Perth Health-preneurs Leading the Charge*, and I was overjoyed to find it was a story of hope, inspiration, and positivity.

It seemed serendipitous that this opportunity had come along, right smack-bang after I'd completed three months alcohol-free. Would this have happened if I'd still been drinking? Did my new clarity and peace of mind attract it somehow?

Whatever the reason, I thanked the Universe profusely. It felt damn good to be a positive influence in the world for once, rather than a destructive force.

~

It took me three more weeks to write the final post in the *100 Days Without a Drink* blog series. The task of articulating the biggest lessons and discoveries felt overwhelming. Where to begin?

Finally, after procrastinating for long enough, I sat down to write. I shared how much healthier I felt. How, after decades of insomnia, I now slept like an angel. How it felt heavenly to wake up every morning with clarity, a feeling of connection, and a sense of purpose. That my face and eyes were less puffy, my skin less dry, and my little wine pouch belly had disappeared.

I wrote about how I felt happier, and more myself than I had in a very long time. About having so much precious time and energy, without late nights or days wasted in hangover-mode. Time for movies (and remembering the entire plot), farmers markets, brunch dates, early morning writing sessions, long walks, new hobbies, and daydreams. Time for greater creativity, productivity, and deep, peaceful relationships.

And I wrote about the part I loved most: the absolute, delicious, blissful *freedom*. Freedom from counting drinks; from giving myself lectures about not making an idiot of myself this time; from saying stupid things I'd regret.

Freedom from believing I could only connect with people when I had a drink in my hand; from searching for late-night cabs in the freezing cold, or worrying about how to get home. Freedom from the morning-after cocktail of tiredness, nausea, anxiety and paranoia.

I was still nervous as I clicked 'publish', but I felt proud of myself. Sobriety wasn't always easy, but it was getting so much easier. And it was so incredibly worth it.

Once again, I received a ton of messages from women around the world, writing things like:

*"Bex, I found your story today and it brought me to tears. It could have been me writing every single word. I am so sick of the hold that alcohol has on me. It's my friend when I'm lonely, when I'm happy, when I'm sad, when something good happens and when something bad happens—but it's not a friend at all. It turns me into a mean person who does ridiculous and hurtful things, it leaves me feeling anxious and sick, and it is a huge waste of time. I'm scared that if I don't stop now, I'm going to destroy my relationships and end up alone forever. I am so glad I found your blog today, it has given me hope."*

*"I am finding this at just the right time! I got really sick after drinking with friends on my 46th birthday last month. I haven't had a drink since, but drinking to excess and being sick has been my M.O. all of my life. I want sober and happy and confident to be my*

*new mode of operation! Thank you, Bex!"*

*"I cannot tell you how much this post meant to me. I too am in the wellness/fitness industry and what you said in response to your client "that's okay" really resonated with me. I have been kicking myself for not practicing what I preach. Thank you for your absolute honesty and inspiration!"*

*"Hi lovely Bex, I think my angels led me to your link, this is precisely what I needed to read at just the right time. It's floored me the parallels between your story and mine, including the health coaching. I feel like such a fraud at times, hating the saboteur within. It's only Day 2 yet I'm feeling good, empowered and a little excited! Your words have really resonated because I can really relate, so thank you for inviting me on the journey of my sober life!"*

# TWELVE

One week after I hit publish on the final instalment of my blog series, I received an email from another journalist:

*Subject: Why Alcohol is Destroying Australians*

*Hi Rebecca,*
*I'm working on a story for The Australian and*
*News.com.au. I'd love to include something from*
*you in this story, as someone who has recently given up*
*alcohol.*
  *What is your experience with alcohol? How did this*
*affect your family/work/health? Why did you decide to*

*stop drinking? How have things changed since then? Do you think the Australian public are aware of just how damaging alcohol can be?*
*Thanks so much, hope to hear from you.*

My initial reaction was nausea. I couldn't decide if it felt like a test, a trap, or just this Universe of ours having a wicked sense of humour and double-daring me.

I wanted to jump at the opportunity to tell my story on a platform like this, with the potential to reach so many more women struggling with the same issues. But at the same time, this was *the largest news publication in the country*. This would be sharing my secret with *the whole world*. Like sailing to a new land and then setting fire to the boat. Yes, this new land appeared to be better, but I'd only been here a few months. What if I wanted to go back?

That night, I drove myself crazy, tossing and turning, unable to sleep.

I thought about the night soon after I'd broken up with my second love, when I met a bunch of friends at my favourite bar. My body had dropped ten kilograms, seemingly overnight. Not wanting to draw attention to it, I dressed in loose clothes, but as my friend Natalie hugged me, she felt straight through the fabric. "Jesus, Bex!" she said, pulling away and holding me at arms length so she could look me up and down. "You're skin and bones."

"Yeah," I shrugged, embarrassed.

"That's it," she said, pulling out her phone. "I'm booking you an appointment with my healer lady."

Her healer specialised in a holistic treatment called Osho Rebalancing; something I'd never heard of. I was apprehensive, but desperate to try anything that didn't involve more hangovers.

"Thank you," I said. "And she'll fix me?"

"No," she said. "She'll help you to fix *yourself*."

Once again, I realised that only I held the power to conquer my fears. No one was going to ride in on a white unicorn to save me.

I thought about all the times I'd been afraid. How I'd stopped eating, stopped breathing, braced my legs so tightly, like I wanted to run away; to escape.

How I drank myself senseless.

In the morning light, I knew it came down to one simple choice.

Love or fear?

*It might not even get published, and if it does, it might not even get read,* I told the beast as it screamed and pounded against my rib cage.

~

"It'll be fine, sweetie, you'll see," Dom said whenever he looked at me. But my mind had a penchant for the dramatic, and my imagination ran wild. "You're damned if you do, and you're damned if you don't!" I babbled, feeling chest pains, I was so stressed out.

The wait was only a few days and yet if felt excruciating. Every time I thought about it, all my original fears threatened to flatten me. The beast licked his lips with glee.

*You're an idiot,* he snarled. *Call the Journalist and tell her to pull the story. You're barely five months sober. Do you really want the whole world to think you have a drinking problem? You don't. Plenty of people love binge-drinking. What if you want to go back to the corporate world? No-one will hire you because they'll think you're an alcoholic, destined to lose the plot at any moment. You'll be branded as diseased and flawed for the rest of your life. You'll never be able to drink again. Is that really what you want? You're fooling yourself if you think coaching clients will want to work with someone like you. No-one will trust you. Dom will leave you, and no-one else will want you. You'll be completely alone.*

Desperately, I searched YouTube for videos of other women telling their story publicly. I needed proof that it was all going to be okay. When I couldn't find any, my mind spiralled out of control. What had I done?

Frozen with fear, I sat in my office chair, staring into space. The beast was right. What did I think I could possibly offer, that would help other people? Receiving a few nice comments on my blog posts was one thing. This was another thing entirely. This was a huge public platform. I was setting fire to my entire business, my reputation, my *life*.

When I didn't come out of the study for lunch, Dom came looking for me.

"You okay?" he asked.

"No," I shook my head, and burst into tears. "I can't do this!" I sobbed.

"Oh, come here," he said, pulling me into a hug. "You can. They need you," he whispered into my hair as he held me. "You're strong enough."

~

Later, keen for any kind of distraction, I busied myself with answering emails. Writing back to the beautiful souls who'd written to me after my latest blog posts helped to calm me down a little.

I'd just finished sending the last message, when a new email appeared my inbox.

> *Subject: Your latest blog posts*
>
> *Hi Bex,*
> *About your latest revelation. I just wanted to con-gratulate you on your courageous decision to admit to being an alcoholic. A life beyond your amazing dreams awaits you in sobriety. Have you been going to AA? There is really nowhere else that can hold someone who is finding their newly sober feet. I've been sober in AA for a number of years. If I can support you in any way, feel free to contact me.*
> *Love and light*

As I read the email, I felt like I'd been slapped in the face. The intention was so kind, and yet...

I stormed into the living room and repeated the email

to Dom. "She thinks I'm an alcoholic!" I spat at him, my inner teenager pitching a fit. Dom just looked at me calmly.

"Do *you* think I'm an alcoholic?" I asked him, my eyes narrowing dangerously. *Daring* him to say it.

He knew better than to step into the ring. "Do *you* think you are?" he asked.

"No!" I yelled, indignation burning my cheeks. I turned and stomped back to the study. For crying out loud! How *dare* they! You can't even *be* an alcoholic unless you drink every day. Everyone knows that! Yes, I always drank more than I meant to, and was almost always the drunkest woman at any given event, but that was just my inner party girl wanting to play. Not an alcoholic who loses her *mind*, for God's sake. Plus, real alcoholics have interventions; all the people in their lives desperately want them to stop drinking. No-one in my life wanted me to stop, besides Dom.

*Because he knows what you know*, a small part of me whispered.

I huffed and puffed for a while longer, but as I began to calm down, something shifted. All those years of shame, of hiding, of not understanding why I could never 'drink like normal people' and not lose my shit. The compulsion, the obsession, the blackouts… What if I was just wired differently?

I'd been addicted to alcohol, just as surely as I'd once been addicted to sugar. That much was clear. So if I wasn't already a full-blown alcoholic, was I destined to become one if I continued drinking? Was I so triggered by this email because it was my every deepest, darkest fear realised?

I certainly didn't feel like I had a fatal *disease*. It sounds ridiculous, but it felt more like a gluten sensitivity. I'd discovered years ago that avoiding gluten altogether was the only way for me to avoid chronic gut pain and eczema break-outs. Ditch gluten, solve the issue. Most people didn't understand this. Well-meaning friends would often urge me to join in, saying, "Oh go on, just have one piece of cake. *Please?* It's my *birthday*." Meanwhile, said friend would be happily getting on with their own life the next day while I was writhing around in agony.

This was so similar, I could barely stand it. Alcohol wasn't good for me. I had two decades of evidence to prove that I was particularly sensitive to it, and that it made me sick physically, mentally, and emotionally. While it was hard to live without gluten—and every time I walked past a bakery rich with the aroma of freshly baked bread, I felt the pang of missing it—my life and health were better without it. The same thing was true of drinking, although of course, worse in this case because alcohol had the added benefit of mind warping, temporary comfort, and escapism.

I thought about a conversation I'd had at lunch a few days earlier with a friend, Maria. She'd always been super healthy and wanted to know more about enrolling in the IIN program.

"I saw your blog posts about sobriety," she said, taking a sip of her fresh juice. "Amazing stuff. You'll drink again eventually, though, won't you?"

"Well, I don't know…" I blushed. *Note to self; must get better at talking about this stuff.*

"But you weren't an alcoholic. What if you have a really stressful day and you just want a lovely glass of red? You can just have one, can't you?"

*See!* The beast screamed in my head. *She's seen you drunk and sloppy a hundred times and she thinks you can have just one. You can just have one!*

"But I don't want just one, Maria," I declared, as much to her as to the beast. "I want ten."

It occurred to me how mixed up we are as a society around alcohol. We'd never urge ex-smokers to 'just have one', because we know they've fought so hard for freedom from their addiction, and that would only be pushing them straight back to square one.

I thought about another recent night, when Dom and I had arrived back at our apartment and I saw that I had a missed call from another friend, Jenny. I called her straight back. "Sorry I missed your call, hon. We were invited to drinks at our neighbour's apartment."

"Huh?" she said. "But you guys don't drink?"

"Yeah," I shrugged and smiled, even though she couldn't see me. "We took our soft drinks."

"Oh my God, they'll think you're alcoholics!" she yelled, before roaring with laughter, making me suspect she'd had a few drinks herself.

"Well, it's only Monday," I protested. "And I told them I'm a health coach."

"Oh, okay," she conceded, when she'd calmed down. "Anyway, about tomorrow…"

Afterwards, I couldn't get the conversation out of my head. How messed up are our ideas about alcohol, if we can't even visit new friends on a Monday night and feel okay about not imbibing? How crazy is it that we still feel peer pressure past the age of seventeen? I'd been a huge part of that culture for so long, but now I was starting to see things differently. On my deathbed, I wondered which one I'd regret more; drinking with everyone else while it tormented me, or honouring the truth. I knew the answer.

I still wasn't convinced that the label of alcoholic was either well defined or helpful, but for the first time in my life, I was no longer afraid of it. Because in the end, it didn't matter whether I drank every day, or binge-drank once a week. What mattered was the effect drinking was having on my soul. Alcohol wasn't good for me and I was much better off without it. People could call that what they liked.

~

A few days later, I was surprised to see an email from an old colleague pop into my inbox:

*Hi Rebecca,*

*Well done on this change in lifestyle for you. Standing up and recognising that you, or anyone else, has a*

*problem is just the first step. You have seen it and done*
*something about it, something that cannot be said for*
*all of us.*
    *Great to see. All the best.*

My stomach lurched and for a second I thought I might throw up. The email seemed innocent enough, except that this guy was trouble with a capital T. In my wilder days, we'd partied together. At first I'd thought he was great fun, but as we'd spent more time together at boozy events, he'd become too wild, even for me. He seemed dangerous and emotionally volatile, prone to fly off the handle at any moment. I quickly ended our friendship, and moved on to other drinking friends.

There were only two ways he could know about this; via my blog, or the newspaper article. As I typed News.com.au into my browser and clicked *enter*, my hands were shaking.

The article flashed onto my screen. It included interviews with three other Australians, their lives all affected by alcohol. The last story was my photo, name, and interview. I read the entire thing without breathing.

It was good. Really good. Thought-provoking and sensitive. An article that could be of great help and hope to many people.

I exhaled and clicked back over to my email inbox. Five new emails waited for me, each with a single subject line: "Thank you".

Inside the long emails, they confided their stories, saying things like:

> *"Thank you for your honesty! I cried as I read your post. It could have been me writing every word."*

> *"Your story stood out to me in particular. It felt like your words were mine. I can't bring myself to talk about this with anyone but myself, I'm too ashamed. I just wanted you to know the impact you made on me just from your contribution to that article, so thank you."*

> *"It felt like it was my story, someone had pinched my thoughts, feelings and eccentricities, and put them on paper without telling me first. Thank you for telling your story. It has made my feel incredibly positive about the changes I have been wanting to make for a long time."*

I also received an email from the journalist, thanking me for my help and including a link to the article. As I hit 'reply' to thank her for such a beautiful article, hot tears stung the back of my eyelids. I thanked the ever-loving sunshine that I hadn't chickened out of contributing to the story.

What if the very thing I believed to be my biggest flaw and weakness, actually turned out to be my biggest gift?

When I began this sobriety challenge, I wondered whether I'd been trapped at the same level of emotional maturity as when I first picked up the bottle. Thinking back over how I handled myself and situations in the past, I could definitely see that sixteen year old in charge.

How remarkable to see that an adult was emerging to step into the drivers seat of my life now. Yes, this road was bumpy, challenging and emotionally exhausting, but it was also reliable, trustworthy, and *real*. I had a feeling I was going to like it here.

I was also beginning to have an idea.

# THIRTEEN

"So, I've been thinking," I announced to Dom over breakfast, finally finding the courage to broach the subject. "Every week, I receive more emails from women asking how I got sober and stayed that way, so they can do it too. But obviously, it's too huge to sum up in an email. So, what if…" I trailed off, feeling shy all of a sudden.

"What if…What?" he prompted.

"Well, what if we created an online coaching program, like The Sparkle Project, but about sobriety instead?" I held my breath as he mulled it over. Part of me hoped he thought it was a terrible idea, so I'd be off the hook. I could go back to being just a regular health and life coach, nice and cozy in my comfort zone.

"I love it," Dom nodded, sipping his coffee. "You could share all the things you did that helped you."

"Exactly," I smiled, surprised to find myself feeling those tingles of nervous excitement I got whenever inspiration struck. "Well, okay then! I guess I'll start jotting down some ideas."

"Go for it," he smiled.

I headed straight for the study. Above all, I knew in my heart that I wanted this program to be about wellness and empowerment. I wanted to help liberate women from fear, or thoughts of being a social outcast, so they could experience for themselves what a huge difference sobriety could make to their lives. And to discover what I did; that the freedom of sobriety felt incredible.

I opened up a large notebook and began brainstorming. On one page, I wrote all the holistic lifestyle elements that had helped me the most, especially during the first few challenging months. On another page, I wrote the bigger picture concepts, like: beautiful, positive, inspiring, and soulful. I wanted to create the kind of program I would have loved, but hadn't been able to find.

~

"So how's the not-drinking thing going?" Sophie asked as we walked around the river.

"Really good. Actually, we're thinking of maybe creating an online coaching program. About sobriety." I looked at her sideways, nervously gauging her reaction. She was the first person in the world I'd mentioned this idea to, besides Dom.

"Oh, wow," she said, breaking into a smile. "That's a brilliant idea!"

"Oh!" I laughed, relieved that she didn't think I was bonkers, and seemed as excited about the idea as I was. "I'm just figuring out the best kind of format. You know, what would be most helpful. In The Sparkle Project, we had weekly modules but I know that early sobriety is so freaking hard, I'm thinking mini daily modules would be better. Something to distract and support them each night at Wine O'Clock."

"Hmmm," she mused. "Maybe you could do something like my running app. So, I want to be able to run half marathons, right? But getting to that level is so daunting. With my app, I check in every day and it just tells me what to do that day. So, at first it was just to run for ten minutes. Then each day, it challenges you a little more, until one day you look up and hey presto, you can run twelve k's!"

"Oh my God, I love that," I breathed. "It makes the whole process less scary. So with *this* program, it would be: how can you take care of yourself a little better today? How can you handle all the crazy emotions? How can you show yourself more love?"

"Exactly," she said with a triumphant grin.

My mind whirred all the way home.

"Want to go for a walk?" I asked Dom, the second I

bounded through the front door.

"Uh… didn't you just go for a long walk?" he asked, baffled.

"Yep! But I've got some ideas!" I whooped, doing a damn fine impression of a cheerleader. We always did our best brainstorming as we walked.

Dom grabbed his shoes and we hit the street.

"How hard is it to make a phone app?" I asked him as soon as we were outside.

"Well… It's more complicated than you might think."

"Oh," I replied, crestfallen.

"But if you make a website that's super mobile-responsive, it's practically an app, anyway. People can still log in and access it every day from their phones. Why's that?"

I told him all about my chat with Sophie.

"I like it," he nodded as he thought it over. "We could create a membership site, like we did for The Sparkle Project, but with daily incremental levels. How many days were you thinking?"

"Well, it took me a good three months to start feeling better. So… ninety days?" I asked, hopeful.

"Okay, so ninety levels. Sounds complicated, but not impossible. I'll start looking into it when we get back."

As we turned and headed for home, a flood of emotions washed over me. Excitement at the possibility of helping other women, like the ones who had written to me. Fear of putting myself out there in this way. Anxiety about whether I had what it took to lead a program like this.

But most of all, I felt like I was meant to do this.

~

"Okay, I can definitely create a membership site with that many levels," Dom confirmed the next day. "So we can go ahead and register a domain if you like, and I can start building it. What do you want to call it?"

Oh, boy. I hadn't thought that far ahead yet. "Hhhmm. Sparkly and Sober?" I suggested.

"No. 'Sparkly' feels too light—too superficial—for this kind of topic."

He was right. "Savvy Sobriety?" I tried again.

"Hmm. It's not quite right," he shook his head. "I know! How about Sexy Sobriety?"

I raised an eyebrow. "I'm not sure I want the word 'sexy' in it."

"Why not?"

"Because… what about trolls, and porn searchers, and stuff? Won't we attract all sorts of weirdness?"

"It'll be fine. Plus, sobriety *is* sexy," he assured me. I thought about all the times I'd been drunk, and how it had made me feel like I was the most powerful seductress in the history of the Universe. In reality, no doubt I'd looked like a drunken buffoon. Sobriety—being completely conscious—really *was* sexy.

"I don't know…" I said, biting my lip.

"Didn't you say that this program is about authentic confidence and empowerment? Well, what's more sexy than that?"

"Well, I guess it's about time sobriety got a make-over."

I nodded slowly, not entirely convinced yet, but warming to the idea. "The 'teetotaller' stereotype is boring and lame."

"There you go," he smiled, already turning back to his desk to get started on designing the logo.

"Okay, let's think it over," I said to his back.

~

"What do you think of this?" Dom asked, turning his computer screen towards me so I could see the 'coming soon' page he'd created. "I know you usually love having a billion colours, but I thought we could try something different this time."

"Oh, wow," I breathed. "I love it." It was modern and sleek, using a clever combination of just black, white, grey, and a bold rose-pink.

"Oh good," he laughed, tilting his screen back.

"Okay, so I've purchased the domain, and registered the business name, so we're full steam ahead," I told him, reading from my to-do list.

"Cool. Hey, why don't you post in the B-School Facebook group about the name and the idea, and see what they think?" he suggested. "It'll be a good way to gauge demand as well. I'll create a section on this page to collect subscribers."

I nodded, thinking it over. B-School was the online business and marketing course I'd taken the year before. The Facebook group was filled with thousands of entrepreneurs. I loved being inspired by the stories they shared in the group, and often read them aloud to Dom. They'd been a huge factor in our original decision to leave the corporate world.

"Okayyyy…" I stalled. Truthfully, the idea scared the crap out of me. Just as with the News.com.au article, it was one thing to talk about the idea with my nearest and dearest. It was another thing entirely to open it up to the scrutiny of thousands of fellow entrepreneurs.

I couldn't bring myself to do it that day. Or the day after that.

Finally, Dom's persistence spurred me into action. I opened the B-School Facebook group, took a deep breath, and typed a post telling them about the idea. I included a link to the page we'd created on the Sexy Sobriety website.

*It's up to you now, Universe,* I thought. *If this is a terrible idea for me to take on—either the program or long-term sobriety—now's your chance.*

No sooner had I hit 'post' with a trembling finger, than the comments of love and support started rolling in. One after another, they wrote things like:

> *"Such a great idea. This will be a great support and reality check for women, and help so many people. Good luck, Bex, and keep us posted on your progress."*

> *"Way to go, Rebecca! If this isn't stepping up, I don't know what is."*

*"Well done, Bex! This is a wonderful story. You've turned your pain into something positive."*

*"Fabulous story. Love the name. Sobriety IS sexy, far more than being face down on the couch looking like you've been dragged through a hedge backwards (experience talking here!). This site is something I will definitely be recommending to clients. Well done on all fronts."*

As I read through them, I felt overwhelmed with emotion. "They love it," I told Dom, attempting to get a hold of myself. I was sure *real* entrepreneurs didn't cry whenever they tested a new idea. "So how many subscribers do we need before we definitely go ahead with the idea?"

"A hundred should do it," he replied.

"A *hundred?*" I spluttered. "But… That's a lot of people!" He'd obviously gone quite mad.

"It'll happen," he shrugged and smiled.

Sure enough, just a few minutes later, subscription notifications began pouring into my inbox. Within twenty-four hours, over a hundred people had subscribed.

"Cool. Let's get to work!" Dom said with a grin.

~

"One year," I whispered sleepily to Dom, as he reached across the bed to switch off the alarm.

"One year," he whispered, pulling me closer.

I snuggled into him, letting the milestone truly sink in. We'd officially been in business for an entire year. It simultaneously felt like an eternity and no time at all.

We'd booked ourselves onto a sunset cruise that night to celebrate. Dom had taken me on one of these river cruises before, surprising me with tickets when we were first dating, and we'd both loved it. Large windows lined both sides of the boat; the sunset sparkling across the water on one side, the city lights twinkling on the other.

On our last cruise, most of my attention had been fixed firmly on the bar. The manipulative beast in my mind was always calculating how many drinks I could get away with. We'd each had three small glasses of wine, and then rather than just sitting back and enjoying the beautiful sunset like a normal person, I'd spent the rest of the cruise desperately plotting how many more drinks I could squeeze in at dinner afterwards.

I'd always believed that alcohol helped me to relax and celebrate, but seriously, what was relaxing about constantly chasing more? What's to celebrate when a toxic substance holds you in such a vice-like grip?

"Here's to our business birthday," Dom said, returning from the bar with two glasses of sparkling mineral water.

"Cheers!" I smiled. It was a milestone we were never sure we'd see. "To our *entrepreneur-versary.*"

"Cheers!" he grinned, clinking his glass against mine.

"It still doesn't feel real."

"Big year, huh?" He motioned for us to face the water so we could enjoy the view while we chatted. I loved these talks. Time sped up when we were working so hard, and it felt good to reflect on all the things we'd done for the first time.

"An insanely huge year. And we did half of it sober," I laughed, "So, there's that." I was just two weeks away from celebrating six months of sobriety.

"I'm so proud of you, you know," he smiled, looking over at me.

"I know, and I love you so much."

"I love you more," he said, and I tried not to think about how differently this could have all turned out if I'd chosen alcohol.

I turned back towards the water. "We held our first live events, and created eBooks…" I trailed off as I tried to remember everything we'd crammed into this crazy year.

"We created The Sparkle Project and ran it three times." Dom chimed in.

"Four," I smiled. We'd relaunched it again that Monday, guiding a new group of women through the program.

"And created a membership site so they could have access, twenty-four-seven," Dom nodded.

"I graduated from IIN, twice! Two courses of study, *done*. And started working for them as a biz mentor."

"And grew an online community," Dom said.

"And made new friends!" I laughed, realising how many beautiful new friendships we'd formed with other bloggers and creatives.

"And now…" he said, looking over at me.

"Sexy Sobriety," we both said at the exact same moment.

I suddenly felt choked with emotion. I turned back towards the water, attempting to get a grip.

As a breeze danced through the boat, I tried to grasp everything that had happened since we'd taken that leap of faith a year ago. We'd worked harder than we'd ever worked in our lives, but it had also been incredibly rewarding, humbling, and fulfilling. There had been tears of frustration and tears of overflowing joy. It'd been all-at-once insanely confronting, maddening, thrilling, and awe-inspiring.

I'd never expected entrepreneurship and sobriety to actually be crash courses in personal development and emotional maturity. To tackle them at the same time, well, I felt like I could do *anything*. All the ducking and weaving in my past—avoiding memories and parts of myself—it was all beginning to fade away. In its place, was the most delicious feeling; being able to trust and take care of myself.

I was still nervous as hell about the idea of creating a sobriety coaching program, but something within me urged me to keep going. I only hoped that 'something' stuck around.

# FOURTEEN

The next day, before I lost my nerve, I wrote a newsletter to my Vegan Sparkles subscribers and included a link to the Sexy Sobriety webpage. Again, I was nervous as I hit 'send'. So many of the IIN students I mentored each week were on my mailing list, too. What would they think about this new direction? What would IIN think?

Again, I needn't have worried. The subscriptions and love notes poured in.

I showed them to Dom. "Okay, let's kick it up a notch," he said, hugging me. "So, what sort of content do you want to put into the program?"

"Okay, I want to include some recipes," I told him. "Alcohol-free drinks that are sugar-free, sophisticated and fun. Plus, some raw dessert recipes because it's so easy to fall into the sugar trap." I paused, thinking. "Lists, of course," I smiled. He knew how much of a list geek I was. "And downloadable journals, so they can explore what's going on for them. Also, audio pep talks."

I bit the lid of my pen. "Ummm, what else? You know what I would have loved? Interviews with strong, sober women. It's so hard to face this issue when you feel like the only one, or the only stories you hear are about people who miserably white-knuckle it and pine for alcohol for the rest of their lives. Where are all the sexy role models?"

"B-School?" Dom suggested.

"Oh my God," I smiled. "Yes! What better place to find kick-ass babes who've done amazing things in their lives since ditching the drink? You're a genius!" I kissed his lips and skipped to the study, leaving him to order a professional lighting kit, and research how to record video calls.

I sat down at my laptop, swallowed my nerves, and reached out to the B-School Alumni Facebook group again. Surely some of these women had also struggled to put down the glass? I began typing a call-out to anyone who'd love to share their story. I linked to our webpage, just in case they hadn't seen my original post. And with a deep breath, hit 'publish'.

Once again, the love and support flowed in. Best of all, so did the interview bookings.

~

I began the interviews the very next Monday. "Okay, I've got three scheduled today," I told Dom, early that morning.

"Excellent," he said as he set up the room with our new studio lights and microphone.

"I'm a bit nervous," I admitted. It was the first time I'd interviewed other people, and certainly the first time I'd ever asked anyone about their sobriety journey. I was tingling with anticipation, but also unsure of what to expect.

The first three brave women were from the United States, Germany, and England. As they shared their stories, I was struck by how different they were. And yet, at their essence, they were very much the same. We all want to be happy. We all crave connection, peace, and love. We all want to make the most of this precious lifetime.

As I switched off my computer, I sat in silence for a moment, blown away. I was so moved by their tales of heartbreak and triumph.

"How was it?" Dom asked, coming in to the study to shut down the lights.

"Amazing," I breathed. "Incredible. You know, it's one thing to read a woman's story in a book or blog post. It's another thing altogether to have a front row seat as she tells you her story in her own words, tears, smiles, and all."

"So does that mean… Do you want to make the interviews a bigger part of the program?"

"I think they need to be," I nodded as I thought it over. "They're so moving and inspiring. Like, I actually feel newly inspired to continue on my *own* sober journey." I smiled at him. "And I would have *loved* hearing these kinds of stories in my first few months. It feels like such a precious gift to be able to share."

"Okay, let's schedule more interviews," he smiled.

~

When I'd finished recording all the initial interviews, I posted another shout-out in the B-School Facebook group. Many of the original women I'd interviewed chimed in on the post, sharing what a great experience it had been for them, and encouraging others to share their story as well.

Some women booked interview spots, but then pulled out, confiding that they were scared of the stigma if they told their story publicly. I completely understood, but at the same time I felt sad about the shame and secrecy that robs us of our voice.

Other women were excited to hear about the program and thrilled to be able to share their experience to help others.

"Most of them have said to me; I'm so glad someone is doing this, and I'm so glad it's not me," I told Dom after the sixth interviewee had told me exactly the same thing.

"But you want to do it, don't you?" Dom checked, and I loved him for it.

"I do," I nodded. "It's just… They freaked me out a little bit, like they know something I don't. And I just really hope I'm not going to regret going down this path."

"You won't," he reassured me. "It's a bold move, sweetie, but one you're ready for."

I hoped so.

~

The next few weeks passed in a whirlwind of work. Dom continued to build the website, edit the video interviews, and create graphics and downloadable journals. Meanwhile, I continued to record more interviews, create daily articles and activities, record pep talks, and invent new mocktail recipes.

"Come in for an appointment," our Accountant wrote casually in an email one day. "Let's chat about how things are going."

We hadn't been to see him since we'd started our business. We weren't overly concerned about receiving a tax bill—so far our business revenue and expenses barely broke even—and we were still living very modestly on what was left of our savings. But we were nervous about showing him the financial reporting we'd attempted to complete ourselves. We'd spent hours pouring over receipts, and trying to understand the tax jargon on the government website. Each month I reserved two full days to complete and file our statements, and those days drove me nuts.

"Excellent. So what have we got here?" he said, reviewing our statements as we finally sat before him. "Okay, so it looks like The Sparkle Project is coming along nicely. And the IIN coaching. And you've got more clients coming in, Dominic." He looked up at us. "So you're going to focus on ramping up all of these things going forward?"

"Well, actually," I said, pausing to look at Dom for reassurance. He gave a slight nod, so I continued. "We're creating a new program."

"Okay…" our Accountant said slowly, giving me the distinct impression he thought our time would be better spent focusing on the things we'd already created. "So, another one like The Sparkle Project?"

"No, quite different. So we've just registered a new business name for it."

"You have? Okay, let's make sure you've allocated it correctly under your ABN," he said, swivelling in his chair and tapping on his keyboard. "Okay, what's the name?" he asked.

"Sexy Sobriety," I mumbled, leaning over to look at his computer screen so I didn't have to look directly at him.

"Sobriety? Like, not drinking?"

"Uh huh," I nodded, squirming. "It's a sobriety program."

"Right…" he said, swivelling his chair back to face me. "I mean, do you really have time to create another program?"

"Well, we've been working crazy long hours, and it'd definitely be easier not to," I admitted. "But I just feel like this is something I need to do, you know?"

He stared at me for a long moment. "Okay," he shrugged, with a look that said, *It's your funeral.*

I looked at Dom. He smiled at me in reassurance. I

pulled a face and he mouthed, *It's okay.*

In the car on the way home, I was quiet.

"He hasn't seen it from the inside like we have," Dom said, reading my mind. "He doesn't know how many women want and need this."

I nodded, thinking of the emails I'd received, and how much I wanted to share what I'd learnt.

"Okay, so maybe it's not the smartest move, financially," Dom conceded. "Marketing what we've already created would be the easy move, but we're doing something *meaningful* here."

I nodded again. My heart knew he was right. And yet, it wasn't too late to pull out. We'd poured four weeks of work into this project but there'd be hundreds more hours required before we were done. We could easily change direction and work on something else. Expand what we'd already created. Choose something easier.

Going ahead with this plan would mean forever tying my name to sobriety. Was I really up for that kind of commitment? Another six months of sobriety? Twelve months? *Forever?*

My heart whispered yes, while the beast continued to throw a disgusting tantrum in my head.

~

When my phone buzzed one morning, I was delighted to find a text message from Chloé. We'd been working so much that we hadn't seen any of our friends for weeks.

I flicked the message open and read, "Oh my God, Bex! So proud of you!" On my screen was a photo of a page from a newspaper, and right there in the middle of it was a picture of me. *What?*

Shaking, I messaged her straight back, "Oh holy crap! They didn't tell me it made the cut. WOW! Thanks so much, honey! I'm off to buy the paper right now."

A split second later, my phone buzzed again, "YAY! Top Key Influencer, Bex! Amazing!"

A couple of weeks earlier, a reporter from The West Australian Newspaper had contacted me. He told me he was writing a story about social media influencers and wanted to ask me a few questions. I happily answered them, but wasn't quite clear about the direction of the story, and since we were still working twelve hours a day, I hadn't had the time to really think about it.

"Dom!" I bellowed from the study. "Let's take a break!"

I was trembling as we ran to the local newsagency to buy a copy of the paper. We flipped to the Business section, and sure enough, there was my photo and name. I was listed as one of 'Perth's 10 Key Influencers' in Marketing and Media, right next to some of the biggest names in sports and entertainment.

"Wow!" Dom chuckled. I just stared at him, speechless.

"Oh, come here," he said, seeing my eyes fill with tears. He grabbed my hand and guided me over to sit at a nearby café table. I was too choked up to thank him.

I was so surprised when my Vegan Sparkles blog began to grow an audience three years earlier. And now, *this*. Listed as one of the top influencers in my home city of more than two million people. *Was this real life?*

I was a little freaked out about the increased exposure, and all those fears about creating a program about sobriety reared their ugly heads again. But if this was true—if I really was influencing people—I wanted to be sure as hell that I was being a *good* influence. I felt that deep calling rise up again from my soul, urging me to use whatever platform I had to help women get their sparkle back and create a life they loved.

When I got home and checked our Sexy Sobriety Facebook page, I discovered that we'd reached one hundred followers.

This day felt like another huge sign that I was on the right path. *Thank you, Universe.*

# FIFTEEN

Three weeks later, on a Saturday afternoon in late October, I was due to meet five of my girlfriends at a fancy, inner-city hotel. We hadn't caught up in so long, Cara had taken charge and organised a high tea afternoon for us.

Despite my new mission, in the weeks leading up to this date, I'd felt nervous. This wasn't just a 'cake and scones' high tea; this event included champagne. I'd already prepped myself to ask for sparkling water with lemon, but I was worried about how it would feel to be out with my girls again and be the only one not drinking.

Back when we used to hit the town every Friday night, I always planned elaborate agendas, devised to keep them out drinking with me as late as possible.

Today they'd be seeing a very different Bex. Would they implore me to drink with them, telling me this sobriety thing had gone far enough? Would they think I was completely boring? I assumed they hadn't seen each other either for weeks, but what if they had? What if they'd been out every Friday night and had a ton of adventures to talk about, and I felt lame and boring and left out?

The beast had a field day in my mind, reinforcing every fear that popped into it.

Funnily enough, now that the day had arrived, my nerves had all but disappeared. As I did my hair and make-up and chose which outfit to wear, I felt only butterflies of excitement. I couldn't wait to squeeze them all and find out what they'd been up to.

Dom offered to drive me to the hotel, and after I kissed him goodbye, I had to stop myself from blissfully skipping into the foyer. It was a beautiful day, it felt heavenly to dress up after months of working in yoga pants, and I was about to see my girlfriends. Life was good.

"Welcome, ma'am. Do you have a reservation?" the maître d' asked as I entered the restaurant.

"Yes!" I practically sang, giving him Cara's name.

He checked his computer for a moment. "Follow me," he instructed, and proceeded to lead me through the main dining room. The walls danced with light, as crystal glasses reflected chandeliers.

Most of my dining out over the past few months had been in health cafés. I loved the food, but it felt so nice to be somewhere that actually had *tablecloths*. I smiled at the other diners as we walked past.

"Here we are," he said, opening the door to a small, private dining room. It was gorgeous. Beautiful paintings in elaborate gold frames lined the walls, and another huge crystal chandelier sparkled around the room.

My smile grew wider. "Thank you so much," I said, as he left the room.

Cara and Melissa were already seated. "Honeys!" I squealed, as we hugged hello.

The next few hours flew by. The food was delicious, and the stories were so plentiful and hilarious that I found myself frequently crying with laughter. Everyone had been so busy lately, and it was a beautiful afternoon of catching up.

"Is anyone kicking on afterwards?" Cara asked later, as we were getting ready to leave.

I held my breath, not sure how I'd feel if everyone went on to a bar without me, and yet, at the same time, not wanting to go there myself. I wanted to end the day on a high note, dammit.

"Not me," Ashleigh said. "I drove. Plus, I've got stuff to do tomorrow morning."

Then a chorus of similar replies.

Wow. Everyone else really *had* grown up. I imagined what my reaction would have been if I was still drinking. Most likely, I would have taken Cara up on the offer, going extra wild to make up for all my 'boring' friends who went home. For sure, the drinking would have continued when I got home. Cue sloppy and messy Bex, arguments, and hangovers. The same old record I'd been playing for the past twenty years.

As we gathered our things to walk out, I felt an overwhelming combination of relief, gratitude, and humble pie.

"Oh, you're not having more champagne?" the maître d' asked, as we passed back through the main dining room. "Would you like to move to the bar?"

"No, we're with Miss Sexy Sobriety," Meghan said, even though that wasn't the reason. She smiled and winked at me. The title felt *good*.

~

Two days later, I told Sophie about it as we walked around the river. "I actually felt that tingle of excitement before I went out," I babbled. "And I wasn't sure I'd ever feel that again."

"It definitely has to do with mindset," Sophie nodded.

"It does!" I was thrilled that she understood. "I went to the event feeling excited about the location and catching up with everyone, rather than focusing on the drink. And because we hadn't seen each other for a while, there was so much to catch up on, so it just felt exciting. Plus, we were in such a gorgeous room, and I'm sure that helped," I laughed, examining every moment of the event, wanting to capture the feeling in a jar and keep it forever.

"Yep, I think sometimes we drank more because the other people or events were boring," Sophie said.

"Yes," I nodded. "I'm starting to see that. I'm starting to feel like it's okay to skip certain events, *especially* now that the alcohol isn't there as a buffer. Completely sober, I'm more sensitive to loud, rowdy places, and it's just exhausting. I used to want to stay out all night, but now after two or three hours, I've had enough."

"I totally get that," Sophie said. "Especially if you have to talk to a lot of people that you don't know. When I go to work functions and networking things, two hours later, I'm done. I think two hours is my limit on making small talk."

I giggled my agreement. "I need to write all of this into the program," I said, my mind whirling. "It seems so obvious, and yet, when you've been a social butterfly for so many years, you lose your event logic somehow."

I thought about the multitude of times I'd been out and people had left early. "Boring!" I'd yelled, to anyone who would listen.

Not boring, I realised now. *Sane.*

The minute I got home, I recorded a pep talk for the program, covering everything Sophie and I had talked about. High on a wave of inspiration, I also wrote a 'How to Handle Events' guide.

~

My smugness was short-lived. The following week presented the biggest challenge I'd faced in months—possibly for the entire year—a large, formal wedding. Ben and Alana were back from their travels and ready to tie the knot in a huge affair, with close to two hundred guests and a celebration spanning eight hours.

*So much for the two-hour rule.*

I started the day feeling optimistic. I mean, I'd killed it at the high tea. I was almost eight months sober. I'd committed to creating a sobriety program. I'd shared my story publicly. How hard could this really be?

Dom was a groomsman, so he'd be sitting on a separate table to me, but I knew a few of the other guests, so I told myself I'd be fine. But just to be sure, I reviewed the 'handing events' list I'd made a week earlier. I was determined to get through this mammoth event with my sanity intact.

I made a sublime plan for the next morning—a brunch date with a girlfriend—so I had something to really look forward to. In my gratitude journal, I wrote all the good things I was looking forward to at the event. The beautiful venue; the food; being able to catch up with friends; having the chance to dress up; being able to drive myself home like a sober rockstar. I made a batch of raw chocolate desserts so they'd be waiting for me in the freezer when I got home. I put fresh sheets on the bed, and placed a new essential oil and a great book on my bedside table.

Above all, I reminded myself to be patient and kind. *Learning to love events when you're sober takes time,* I told my reflection in the mirror. I repeated a quote I loved from one of my business mentors; *It's always awkward before it's elegant.*

The ceremony took place in a large church. Sunshine

streamed through the stained glass windows, reflecting prisms of coloured light around the sandstone walls. I found a seat along one of the long wooden pews. As the groom's family began to sing hymns, I thought about how truly blessed I was to be there; sober, present, and in love. Dom looked so handsome, standing at the front in his new suit, and my heart swelled with love for him.

I'd had a choice eight months ago; alcohol and a sick relationship with the addict voice in my head, or a beautiful relationship with this incredible man—the love of my life. This all could have ended so differently. Instead, here I was, sitting in the pews, wearing a gorgeous dress, watching my love's best friend get married.

Before I knew it, the entire church full of guests were on their feet, applauding the first kiss of the newly married couple.

We followed the bridal couple outside, mingling and offering hugs and congratulations. Dom pulled me into a few quick happy snaps before the official photographer rounded him up with the bridal party and whisked them away for the formal shoot. Dom's other best friend, Anthony, was also a groomsman. His girlfriend, Sarah, was one of the few other guests I knew.

"Would you like a lift?" I asked her. "I'm driving." As I said the words, I realised how strange they still sounded to my own ears. *Me*, driving at a wedding. Wonders would never cease.

The reception began with a cocktail party in the function room just outside the large ballroom where the dinner celebration was to be held. It was beautiful, with two walls made completely of glass, overlooking the gardens. The other walls were lined with rich mahogany and decorated with elegant frames featuring historic plaques and photos.

At first, I felt confident and proud of myself, acting like a lady at last, rather than pouring free champagne down my throat. But after an hour or so of making small talk and sipping soda water, fatigue began to set in. My feet ached from my high heels, and everyone's excited chatter created a low roar that wore me down. I was disappointed that I wasn't loving this as much as the high tea event, but I consoled myself with the fact that we'd be sitting down soon, and the energy would change.

Another hour later, I swooned with relief as waiters finally swung open the ballroom doors and invited us to find our seats. I was placed on one of the large round tables towards the back of the room, with my friends Thomas and Alice on my left, and a couple I didn't know on my right. There were still at least five hours until midnight, so I prayed they'd be chatty and funny.

Each table was lined with empty wine glasses and bottles of red and white. As we sat down, waiters swiftly placed a full glass of champagne in front of each guest. I didn't have a chance to refuse before I found one in front of me. *Great.*

"I already poured you one," I heard Alice say to Thomas.

"Oh. Well, I'll just put this one aside and drink it later," Thomas laughed, placing his full glass of wine directly in front of me.

So now I had *two* drinks in front of me. *Wonderful.* I tried not to grind my teeth.

Everyone at our table was growing quite tipsy, and although I was now sitting down, I felt even more weary.

*Five hours,* the beast grumbled. *Why are you making life so hard for yourself? Just drink one of them, for God's sake. It's just one drink. What does it matter? Who will care?*

*I will care, that's who,* I retaliated in my head. *Dom will care. My clients will care.*

The beast snarled, *Seriously, you're never going to drink again? There'll be plenty more weddings like this. And dinners, and birthdays, and hens parties, and sundowners. Never again?*

Suddenly, I felt like crying. I attempted to distract myself by joining in the conversation to my left, but they were talking about some great wine bar they'd been to the night before, and everything they'd eaten and drank there. The guests in the seats to my right had just left to mingle with other people. Dom and the bridal party hadn't arrived yet, and I couldn't see anyone else I knew. I wished this didn't feel so hard, but the fact was, I'd had decades of experience socialising whilst drinking, but only eight months experience doing the whole thing sober.

In desperation, I gathered my purse and took myself to the ladies bathroom.

For a moment, as the click-clack of my heels echoed across the whisper-quiet foyer, I contemplated leaving altogether. My keys were in my purse, and our car was parked right outside. Dom could celebrate with his friends and I could pick him up when it finished. Why was I putting myself through all of this, anyway? I knew that big, boozy affairs—especially events where I barely knew anyone—would be easier to tackle when I'd been sober for longer. It was too soon and too dangerous. One wrong move and everything we'd worked so hard for could be destroyed in a single night.

Three women walked into the foyer, interrupting my thoughts. They were having a heated discussion about something, so I quickly ducked around the corner, finding the ladies bathroom. The silence was heavenly. I looked at myself in the mirror and thought about all my reasons for not drinking. This day was about love, family, and friendship, not about me and the beast in my head. Yes, it was challenging, and I felt incredibly emotional, but I imagined being the kind of woman who could have fun sober, no matter what. Authentic playfulness, no toxic substance required. I wanted to be her, more than I wanted to drink.

I took a deep breath and willed myself back to my table, just minutes before the bridal party made their grand entrance.

After an initial group dance, a waiter came over and leant down to speak into my ear. "Excuse me, Miss, would you like to come and join the bridal table?" Confused, I looked over to see Dom and the bride both waving me over. Gratitude washed over me and I bit my lip to stop myself from bursting into tears. Kindness always made me cry.

As the waiter arranged a chair for me, Dom hugged me closer to him, and I felt sweet relief that I hadn't hightailed it outta' there. I wanted to be here for him, not waiting it out alone at home.

A woman plopped herself down into the empty seat beside me.

"Are you Vegan Sparkles?" she asked, wide-eyed with excitement.

"Oh," I laughed as I turned to face her. "I am."

"I love your emails!" she said. "And your website, and I made one of your recipes last week. The laksa. Oh my goodness, it was so good. And now you're creating a sobriety program or something? Tell me about that."

Before I had a chance to answer, she blurted, "Oh, and I'm Nadia, by the way."

We both laughed, and I told her about the program.

"Wow," she said. "I'm a psychologist and I just think it's a fabulous idea that can help so many women. When will it be ready?"

"Thank you so much!" I smiled. The Universe was at it again, spearing signs at my head. "We've been working around the clock to get it finished and we're aiming to launch any day now."

"Like, this week?" she asked.

"Fingers crossed."

The rest of the night passed more quickly. Once I relaxed, I actually had a whole heap of fun. The speeches were hilarious, dinner was delicious, and Dom and I even pulled a few moves on the dance floor.

"So? How was it?" Dom asked later, as we walked to the car.

I squeezed his hand and smiled. "It was the final frontier, and I was triumphant!"

In bed that night, I wrote pages of notes about the experience that I wanted to share with our upcoming Sexy Sobriety members.

"I think we should include live coaching calls in the program," I mumbled sleepily to Dom, reaching over to put my notebook and pen on the bedside table. "Like video calls, so I can share how I handled the most challenging parts of sobriety, and they can ask questions in real-time."

"Sounds like a great idea," he yawned, switching off the light.

As I snuggled down into our soft, comfy bed, I couldn't wait for Launch Day.

~

The following Friday, on November 7th, eight months into my sobriety, it was done. After months of hard work, we finished the membership site, and launched Sexy Sobriety into the world.

"We did it!" Dom laughed, pulling me into a hug.

I could only laugh and hug him back. Sexy Sobriety's doors were open. She was finally here. It still didn't seem real.

"Come on, let's go get some lunch to celebrate," Dom said, still grinning.

"Yes!" I nodded, grinning back. "Actually, just give me a minute."

I couldn't let this milestone pass without one final entry in my gratitude journal.

I strode to my desk and pulled out my gold notebook. Wiping away messy, happy tears, I wrote:

*Thank you, you crazy Universe, for sending me on this insane journey.*

*I finally feel like the confident, empowered woman I always hoped I'd be.*

*With love, and so much gratitude,*
*Rebecca Weller*
*Health Coach. Life Coach.*

I paused for a moment before adding two more words:

*Sobriety Coach.*

# LOVE NOTE

Naturally, the process of writing this book got me thinking about courage, taking risks, and being present for incredible opportunities. I know I wouldn't have had the backbone to embark on a project like this if I hadn't stopped drinking and started looking after myself.

In doing so, I've had the pleasure of meeting incredible women like our beautiful interviewees, and welcoming and supporting thousands of Sexy Sobriety members from around the globe.

Your story doesn't have to be anything like mine. The only question that really matters is: does drinking make you happy? Deep down, does it fill you with joy, or does it feel like it's taking more away from your life than it's giving? If you're completely honest with yourself, do you feel like alcohol is impacting your relationships, self-worth, career, creativity, or health in a negative way?

If so, maybe it's time to try a sobriety experiment of your own. Take sobriety for a test drive. See what life might be like on the sober side.

Because we know what life is like when we're drinking. The hangovers, the shame, the regret, the self-hatred, the destruction.

What we don't know is life sober. And don't you want to see what happens?

Before I stopped drinking, I remember desperately wanting to know what sobriety would be like. What three months was like. What six months was like.

Well, I can't tell you what three years is like (yet), but I can tell you what two years and four months is like. It's like freedom. Exactly like freedom.

I wish you all the health and happiness in the world, beautiful. You deserve nothing less.

With love,
Bex

# ABOUT THE AUTHOR

Rebecca Weller is a Health and Life Coach, Author and Speaker. Named 'one of Perth's leading Healthpreneurs' by The Sunday Times Magazine, Rebecca helps women from around the world to get their sparkle back and create a life they love.

Author of the bestselling sobriety memoir, *A Happier Hour*, *Up All Day, Chameleon: Confessions of a Former People-Pleaser*, and many more, Rebecca writes about love, life, and the strength and potential of the human spirit.

Her work has been featured by The Telstra Business Awards, The Australian, The Huffington Post, MindBodyGreen, Fast Company, Good Health Magazine, Marie Claire Australia, and Elle Quebec.

Rebecca lives in sunny Perth, Western Australia, with her husband, Dominic.

Learn more, plus receive a weekly love note full of inspiration and special bonus gifts, at **BexWeller.com**.

Learn more about Sexy Sobriety:
**SexySobriety.com.au**

Collect your free elixir recipes and Book Club questions:
**SexySobriety.com.au/Book-Bonus**

Read more about sobriety, plus Bex's health coaching studies and experience with IIN:
**BexWeller.com**

# OTHER BOOKS BY REBECCA WELLER

## Up All Day

*What does it take to stay sober long-term?*

*Up All Day* is an uplifting true story about overcoming our limiting beliefs and embracing our dreams - especially when they appear in a form we didn't expect. It's about being brave, and doing hard things (even if you might fail), because of how they *change* you.

## Chameleon: Confessions of a Former People-Pleaser

*What fears and behaviours actually drive our drinking?*

*Chameleon: Confessions of a Former People-Pleaser* is a book about the danger of giving our power away to others, and the magic of finding our way back to ourselves.
In this book, Rebecca explores the many earnest, humiliating – and ultimately liberating – lessons along the way, and how each of us can begin to build a deep and unshakeable confidence.

**Find these, and many more, at BexWeller.com/Books**

www.ingramcontent.com/pod-product-compliance
Lightning Source LLC
Chambersburg PA
CBHW021541260326
41914CB00001B/110